"*10 Simple Solutions to Migraines* is truly a remarkable book that stands apart from the p   d-
aches. I commend her on w   e,
and useful book and know i   <-
ing for meaningful help in e

D0000200

      —*Roger K. Cady, MD,*   *)e*
      Care Center in the Primary Care Network

"Migraine is a complex neurobiological disorder. How can one best manage it? Dawn Marcus has provided ten simple solutions to managing migraines. Her new book will help migraine sufferers get a better handle on their migraine attacks; it also provides a thoughtful, step-by-step approach to cooperative management by patients and their headache care providers."

      —*Stephen Silberstein, MD, president of the American Headache Society*

"An informed patient is an empowered patient. The practical information contained in *10 Simple Solutions to Migraines* will enable you to be an active partner in your healthcare. Learning what triggers your migraine, easy lifestyle changes and how to effectively communicate with your healthcare provider will equip you with better ways to control your migraines and regain your quality of life."

      —*Suzanne E. Simons, executive director of the National Headache Foundation*

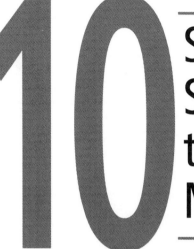

Simple
Solutions
to
Migraines

Recognize Triggers,
Control Symptoms, and
Reclaim Your Life

DAWN A. MARCUS, MD

New Harbinger Publications, Inc.

Publisher's Note

Distributed in Canada by Raincoast Books.

Copyright © 2006 by Dawn Marcus
New Harbinger Publications, Inc.
5674 Shattuck Avenue
Oakland, CA 94609

Cover design by Amy Shoup; Cover image by James Urbach/Superstock; Acquired by Melissa Kirk; Edited by Jessica Beebe;
Text design by Tracy Carlson

All Rights Reserved
Printed in the United States of America

Library of Congress Cataloging-in-Publication Data

Marcus, Dawn A.
  10 simple solutions to migraines : recognize triggers, control symptoms, and reclaim your life / Dawn A. Marcus.
        p. cm.
  ISBN-13: 978-1-57224-441-2
  ISBN-10: 1-57224-441-0
  1. Migraine—Treatment. 2. Headache—Treatment. I. Title: Ten simple solutions to migraines. II. Title.
  RC392.M37 2006
  616.8'4912—dc22

                                                    2006002531

New Harbinger Publications' Web site address: www.newharbinger.com

08 07 06

10 9 8 7 6 5 4 3 2 1

First printing

Contents

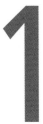

Understand Your Migraine

For years, I've been trying to keep up my professional life in spite of my headaches. My doctor said the headaches are probably from work stress, but I even get them on weekends and vacations. I've tried several medications, but nothing seems to help. I miss family and social events, and I even lost a work promotion. I feel like these headaches are controlling my life.

Untreated migraine can seem to control your life—dictating if you can go to work or a child's soccer game, limiting what foods you can eat, and causing frustration and depression. The good news for migraine sufferers is that there are a lot of effective treatments available to help prevent and treat headaches. Unfortunately, there is no quick fix or simple cure for migraines. With education and consistent application of headache management techniques, most migraine sufferers can significantly reduce their headaches and the impact migraine has on their lives.

How Do You Know It's Migraine?

There is no X-ray or blood test to identify migraine. Migraine is diagnosed when a person has several of these typical headache features:

- pain on one side of the head.
- pain that feels like a throb or pulse.
- pain that limits activities.
- a need to dim lights or go to a dark room.
- a need to avoid noises or go to a quiet room.
- nausea or vomiting.
- odors like smoke and perfume are nauseating.
- bending over with head between knees worsens pain.

Not everyone with migraine has all of these features. You may have a severe, throbbing pain on both sides of the head that makes you seek a dark, quiet room. Even though the pain affects both sides of the head, most of the headache characteristics are migraine features. You may notice different characteristics with different headache attacks. For example, some migraines may cause throbbing pain and vomiting, while others cause a dull pain without vomiting. Headaches that limit your activities and make you close curtains, turn off the television, and avoid odors are probably also migraines. Remember, you don't have to vomit or even be nauseated for your headache to be a migraine.

What Causes Migraine?

When you see a doctor for migraines, you'll probably hear that "everything looks normal." Your doctor means that you don't have another serious illness, a brain tumor, an aneurysm, or an infection causing the headache. This doesn't mean that migraine is imaginary. It just means that today's tests aren't sensitive enough to find the abnormalities in the body that result in migraine. Research studies have identified several important factors that contribute to migraine, including an inherited headache susceptibility and increased sensitivity of the brain to pain messages.

HEADACHE SUSCEPTIBILITY

Like many health conditions, migraine is probably caused by a combination of genetic and environmental factors. Migraine tends to run in families. About half to two-thirds of *migraineurs* (people with migraine) have close relatives with migraine. Migraine is more likely to run on the mother's side of the family. A study of over 8,000 adult twin pairs found migraine in about 12 percent (Honkasalo et al. 1995). When one twin had migraine, an identical twin (who shares the same genetics) was over twice as likely to also have migraine compared with a nonidentical twin. This study showed that about half the risk for migraine comes from your genes. The other half comes from environmental factors.

So far, studies have not identified a specific gene abnormality that causes most kinds of migraine. *Familial hemiplegic migraine* is a rare type of migraine that has been linked to specific gene abnormalities. People with familial hemiplegic (meaning "half-body paralysis") migraine experience paralysis or weakness over half of the body during migraine attacks. Other family members will have the same type of migraine attacks with paralysis. In these people, genetic mutations have been found on chromosomes number one and nineteen. Although more typical migraine attacks also run in families, these same chromosome abnormalities have not been seen in typical migraineurs.

MIGRAINE TRIGGERS

If you inherited a susceptibility to migraine, a variety of environmental factors may trigger your headache. As you can see from the table, each trigger usually provokes a migraine for only about 10 to 30 percent of people with migraine (Marcus 2003b).

People in Whom Each Trigger Will Usually Provoke a Migraine	
Stress	33 percent
Glare	29 percent
Skipping meals	28 percent
Change in sleep	26 percent
Odors	26 percent
Change in weather	24 percent
Alcohol (for example, red wine)	10 percent
Exercise	10 percent
Caffeine	9 percent
Food	8 percent

Identifying your headache triggers can be difficult because individual triggers don't always provoke a headache and many triggers may occur together. For example, on a stressful day, you may skip lunch and have coffee and a chocolate bar as an afternoon snack. That evening, you get a migraine. What caused the migraine? Was it stress, skipping lunch, caffeine, or chocolate? Probably it was a combination of all of these.

Imagine that you have a scale inside of your head, with one side able to prevent a migraine and the other side provoking it. When enough headache triggers have been added to the headache-provoking pan, the scale tips and you experience a headache. Some people naturally have their scale balanced so that a lot of triggers are needed to provoke a migraine. These people may have to miss a night of sleep, skip breakfast, drink too much caffeine, have a stressful day, and experience a weather change before a migraine occurs. For other people, adding just a couple of factors into the headache pan may be enough to tip the balance of the scale into causing a migraine. Unfortunately, this means you may have to change a variety of environmental and lifestyle factors in order to prevent migraines. Just avoiding a couple of possible triggers may not be adequate. In later chapters, when I discuss trigger avoidance, I'll focus on those triggers that you can change, like your response to stress, scheduling meals and sleep, and proper nutrition.

PHYSIOLOGY OF MIGRAINE

Years ago, doctors believed that migraine was caused by a disorder of blood vessels around the brain. During a migraine, you may notice a throbbing sensation, as if you can feel your heart pounding in your head. You may also notice the blood vessels at your temples become more prominent and tender during a migraine. These changes led doctors to refer to migraine as a *vascular* or blood vessel headache. Today, we know that the blood vessels are only a small part of the story. Migraine is actually caused by interactions among blood vessels, nerves, and muscles. Each of these components makes important contributions to the overall migraine experience.

The brain pumps out several nerve messenger chemicals (including serotonin, norepinephrine, dopamine, GABA or gamma-aminobutyric acid, and nitric oxide) that send pain messages when you're exposed to migraine triggers. These chemicals are normally found in the brain and are important for sending a wide variety of brain messages, including pain and migraine. During a migraine, nerve messengers signal a major pain relay station in the brain, the *trigeminal nucleus* or fifth cranial nerve. This relay station receives nerve signals and redirects them to other brain areas. Signals from the trigeminal nucleus will:

- cause blood vessels around the brain to expand and throb

- signal the brain vomiting center to cause nausea

- increase sensitivity to lights, sounds, and odors

- cause spasm of muscles in the back of the head and neck

- cause the overall experience of head pain

Because the trigeminal relay station controls so many different brain functions, migraine can be fairly complicated, affecting many systems in the body.

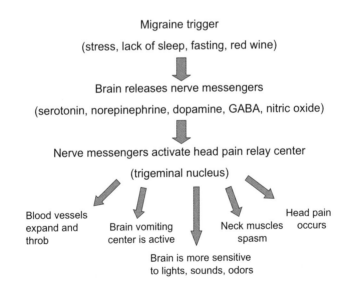

The trigeminal system also causes *allodynia,* or increased sensitivity of the skin during migraine. Allodynia means that touching the skin feels painful. During a migraine, you probably won't say that you have allodynia, but you may feel that your scalp or hair hurts or that it hurts to brush your hair. You may also notice that wearing your glasses or earrings is uncomfortable. Some people mistakenly believe this is because their face is swollen. A small number of migraineurs notice that tight-fitting clothing is uncomfortable during a migraine. All of these changes are symptoms of allodynia. Recognizing allodynia is important because migraine medications work best if they are taken before allodynia occurs.

BRAIN CHANGES WITH MIGRAINE

Because migraine pain can be so disabling, some migraineurs worry that the migraine attacks are causing permanent brain damage. About one-third of migraineurs will have small white spots on magnetic resonance imaging or MRI scans of the brain (Marcus 2003a). In addition, preliminary research has found iron deposits in the brain in some migraine sufferers (Welch et al. 2001). Fortunately, neither of these brain changes seem to be related to any brain damage or loss of intellectual function in migraine patients.

However, having migraine episodes seems to increase the risk for developing future migraines. This is a function of *brain plasticity,* or the ability of the brain to mold or change over time. You experience brain plasticity any time you learn a new skill. For example, it takes a lot of conscious effort when you first learn to write your name, ride a bicycle, or play the piano. The more you practice, the easier these skills become. Eventually, you can write your name effortlessly or ride a bike without even thinking about it.

The same is true with migraines. Every time you have a migraine, your brain is learning more efficient ways to send those migraine messages along the nerves in the brain.

Unfortunately, practice makes perfect for migraine, too. So over years, you may notice your migraines are more frequent or more severe. Or you may notice that you're more sensitive to migraine triggers.

> *I used to be able to stay up all night and skip meals with no problem. Now I get a migraine if I lose a few hours of sleep or miss lunch.*

The good news is that the brain can also effectively learn how to block migraine messages with training. Brain plasticity makes managing migraines particularly important to help reduce future migraine attacks.

NEW RESEARCH ON MIGRAINE CAUSES

A new area of research into the cause of migraine involves looking at the walls that separate the four chambers of the heart. While a fetus is developing, there is a hole in the wall separating the two top chambers of the heart. This hole is called the *foramen ovale* (meaning "oval hole"). This normally closes before birth. For about 20 percent of people, this hole remains open, causing a *patent* (or open) *foramen ovale,* or PFO. When blood returns to the heart from the body, it usually has to pass through the lungs, where toxins are removed and oxygen is put in before the blood travels to the brain and back to the rest of the body. In people with a PFO, the blood can bypass the lungs by crossing through the hole in the wall between the sides of the heart and go straight to the brain and body. Babies with large PFOs may have trouble getting enough oxygen in their blood. Adults with PFOs may develop strokes because small blood clots don't get filtered out by the lungs. Interestingly, patients with migraine with *aura* (changes in vision that sometimes occur before a migraine) are about twice as likely to have a PFO as people with migraine without an aura or people with no migraines (Beda and Gill 2005).

Currently, doctors only look for PFOs or other types of holes between the heart chambers (*atrial septal defects,* or ASDs) in migraine patients who have had unexplained strokes. A special ultrasound test of the heart, a *transesophageal echocardiogram,* watches bubbles as they move through the heart to see if there's a hole in the wall.

Several studies have shown that patients undergoing a repair of a PFO or ASD often experience a marked reduction in the severity and frequency of migraine attacks—both migraine with aura and migraine with no aura (Azarbal et al. 2005; Beda and Gill 2005; Reisman et al. 2005). Researchers speculate that chemicals that would normally be filtered by the lungs may trigger migraines. Another possibility is that there may be a genetic link between heart defects and migraine. Several other studies, however, have reported worsening of migraine or the development of new migraines after these repairs (Beda and Gill 2005; Mortelmans et al. 2005). These studies question the importance of a relationship between migraine and heart defects. Future research studies testing large numbers of migraineurs with PFO or ASD will help clarify this possibly important link.

Not Every Headache Is a Migraine

The first and most important question to ask about headaches is whether you have one or more than one type of headache. For example, Tim has two headaches: a severe throbbing pain with vomiting that sends him to bed in a dark, quiet room once a month, and a milder throbbing pain that makes him nauseated and limits his activities about once a week. In fact, Tim has one type of headache (a migraine) that can be more or less severe. Katie also has two headaches: a severe throbbing pain on one side of the head with her menstrual periods, and a mild, dull squeezing pain across her forehead when work stress is high. She truly has two different types of headache: menstrual migraine and dull tension-type headaches.

In the next chapter, I will review the different features of common nonmigraine headaches, including tension-type headache, medication overuse or rebound headache, post-trauma headache, and cluster headache. It's important to correctly identify the type of headache or headaches that you have to ensure proper treatment. In addition, it's important to know if your headache may be a sign of a more serious health problem.

The following headache characteristics are warning signs that you should see a doctor:

- new headache or change in pattern during the last two years

- pain in the back of the head or neck

- pain with exertion, coughing, sneezing, straining, or during sex

- pain that occurs with changes in posture or when you're lying down

- new headache after age fifty

- other body symptoms besides headache, such as fever, fatigue, joint problems, unintended weight loss, weakness, numbness, or problems with concentration, memory, or vision

These headache features *may* suggest a more serious health problem, but they are often found in patients with typical migraine or other types of headache. You should see your doctor if you develop a new headache or have a change in your headache pattern or responsiveness to previously effective treatment. Headaches caused by other diseases are more likely to develop in older adults, so if you're over age fifty and you develop a new headache, you should see your doctor. Tell your doctor about other new health problems that may have started when the headache began or worsened.

Usually, after an examination, your doctor can reassure you that the headache is not a sign of another medical condition.

How Is Migraine Treated?

While doctors and friends who don't have troublesome headaches may think or say, "So what. It's just a headache," keep in mind that treating migraine is very important. Just suffering through headaches can lead to significant disability, hurting your quality of life, straining your relationships with family and friends, and hindering your ability to work effectively. A survey of twenty-five countries spanning four continents evaluated work disability from migraine (Gerth et al. 2001). The average migraineur lost the equivalent of twenty workdays each year due to migraine from work absence and reduced productivity.

Most migraines can be diagnosed and effectively managed by your family physician or primary care doctor. To identify a doctor in your area with a special interest or expertise in headache management, check with your family doctor or nearby medical school. The American Council for Headache Education Web site (see chapter 10) also provides a list of headache doctors in different cities across the nation.

Migraine treatment includes both nonmedication and medication treatments. Effective nonmedication treatments include stress management, relaxation and biofeedback, and lifestyle modification (such as avoiding fasting and changes in sleep cycles). Moderately effective nonmedication treatments include targeted stretching exercises, dietary restrictions, and some herbal, vitamin, and mineral supplements. Medications are available over the counter and by prescription to treat migraines. Medications include drugs to treat individual migraine attacks (*acute* care) and drugs to reduce the frequency of future migraines (*preventive* care). I will discuss nonmedication and medication acute and preventive therapies in detail in chapters 4 and 5.

Special Issues for Women

My migraines started with my periods when I was thirteen. I thought I was cured when I got pregnant, but the migraines came right back the first week after my baby was born. When I finally reached menopause, I expected my migraines to go away for good. But now I'm getting hot flashes and my migraines are actually worse.

Migraine is about three times more likely to occur in women than in men. Migraine commonly begins in girls the same year they begin to menstruate and changes over the years with hormonal changes:

- Migraine worsens with menses in 60 percent of women.

- Migraine improves with pregnancy in 50 to 60 percent of women.

- Migraine typically worsens during early menopause.

- Migraine improves in over 60 percent of women after natural menopause (Neri et al. 1993).

- Migraine worsens in over 60 percent of women after hysterectomy (Neri et al. 1993).

These changes in women's migraine are often triggered by changing estrogen levels.

In addition to helping girls change into women, estrogen is also an important pain blocker. When estrogen begins to cycle, estrogen is turned on as a pain regulator. This may explain why migraine usually starts in girls at puberty. High estrogen blocks pain, so migraines often improve during the second trimester of pregnancy, when estrogen levels become very high. Low estrogen increases pain messages. So migraines often increase with ovulation, menstruation, and after delivery of a baby, since estrogen levels fall to very low levels at these times. During the early stages of menopause, estrogen levels typically change a lot, often resulting in hot flashes and a worsening of headache. Once women are in later menopause, their estrogen levels are stable, and migraines tend to improve. Curiously, migraine tends to worsen after hysterectomy, so only natural menopause helps improve migraine.

Special Issues for Children

Nine-year-old Steven leaves class during a math test for a "headache." He tells the school nurse his head hurts and puts his hand over his forehead to show her where. Steven takes a Motrin tablet, naps for forty-five minutes, and wakes feeling well and ready to return to class. The nurse concludes, "How convenient. His 'headache' went away as soon as math class was over. And who ever heard of a boy with migraines?"

Headaches in kids and teenagers are often ignored or misinterpreted as excuses to miss stressful or unpleasant activities. Migraine occurs in about 5 to 10 percent of children and adolescents (Özge et al. 2003; Lipton and Bigal 2005). Boys actually are more likely to have migraine before age ten than girls. After puberty, girls have more migraines. The good news for boys is that their migraines often go away by age twenty-five, while girls tend to have migraines until menopause.

Migraine is frequently overlooked in kids because their headaches are different from adults'.

In adults:

- pain is on one side of the head or around an eye
- pain is throbbing or pulsating
- pain typically lasts six to twelve hours
- there is usually nausea, vomiting, or sensitivity to noise and lights

In children:

- pain is on both sides of the head, typically across the forehead
- pain is described as "dull," or kids may simply say that their head "hurts"
- pain typically lasts one to three hours
- there is often no nausea, vomiting, or sensitivity to noise and lights

As in adults, migraine in children is not likely to affect the back of the head. Typically, a child with migraine places her hand on her forehead to show where it hurts. Kids won't usually call their pain throbbing, describe sensitivity to noises or lights, or mention nausea. Even kids who vomit usually don't link vomiting with the migraine. Asking children to draw a picture of what the headache feels like can be an effective way to "see" their migraine symptoms.

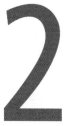

Get a Proper Diagnosis

*I've had headaches since I was a kid. First,
I was told they were "stress" headaches. Later,
my doctor diagnosed migraine. Now I'm seeing a
new doctor who tells me they're cluster headaches.
I don't know what I've got!*

Getting a correct diagnosis is the first step to managing headaches. There are no tests to distinguish among common causes of recurring headaches. X-rays, MRI scans, and blood tests are used to make sure your headache isn't caused by another health problem. These tests usually tell you what you *don't* have: you don't have a brain tumor or an aneurysm. There are no tests to tell you what you *do* have.

Different types of headache are identified when headache features fit into specific patterns. Many people have some features of several different headache types. When many features of a certain headache type occur together, that is probably the correct diagnosis. Understanding those headache features your doctor uses to assign a headache diagnosis will help you to better monitor your own headaches for these characteristics. This will allow you to provide good information to your doctor to ensure an accurate diagnosis.

In this chapter, I'll describe several types of headache: migraine, medication overuse headache, tension-type headache, post-trauma headache, cluster headache, and sinus headache. After each different headache is described, you can take a short quiz to help you decide if you have that type of headache. If you have more than one type of headache, pick your most severe and mildest headaches and take each quiz twice: once for each type of headache. This way, you'll be able to decide if you have one type of headache (such as migraines that are both mild and severe) or two types of headache (such as migraine plus tension-type headache). Remember, these quizzes are designed to help you identify headaches that you have had chronically. See your doctor if you develop a new type of headache.

When Should You See Your Doctor?

Discuss your headaches with your doctor to get a positive diagnosis. You should see your doctor when:

- you're not sure of your headache diagnosis

- your headaches have changed

- you develop a new type of headache

- your headache treatment isn't working

Your doctor will need to know your headache characteristics to make a diagnosis.

- How often do you have a headache?

- What does it feel like?

- Does anything else bother you during the headache besides pain?

- What medications are you using for your headache?

- Do you have any other health problems?

Review the characteristics of the common headaches listed in this chapter to help you recognize your own headache pattern. To help your doctor make your headache diagnosis, share the results of these headache quizzes.

Recognize Typical Features of Migraine

My mom gets a migraine with her menstrual periods. She goes to bed and puts a washcloth over her eyes and forehead, and she can't stand noise or lights. Even smells bother her. About half of the time she vomits, which makes the headache better. I get a headache about once a week that starts in my temple and then affects my whole head. I never miss work, but I'm less productive. I try to turn down the radio and lights. I never vomit.

People often say, "My mom gets terrible migraines, but I just have a regular headache." Unfortunately, not recognizing these "regular" headaches as migraines may prevent people from getting effective treatment. Migraines aren't always the same for everyone, even among family members.

MIGRAINE CHARACTERISTICS

Migraine pain is often focused on one side of the head. During a migraine, pain can start on one side before affecting the whole head, or it can move from the whole head to just one side. Pain may also switch sides during a migraine. Your headache is considered to be *unilateral*, or one-sided, if the pain is focused on one side of the head at some time during the headache rather than always on both sides at the same time or across the forehead.

Migraine is usually best diagnosed by your behavior during a headache. During a migraine, people often:

- go to a dark, quiet room

- avoid other people

- need to avoid glare, smells, and smoke

- put a washcloth over the forehead or eyes

- lie down quietly

- cut back on work or other activities

Without treatment, migraine attacks usually last about six to twelve hours. In some people, migraines may resolve more quickly, or they may last for one or more days. When a migraine is over, you may feel temporarily hungover. Then you'll be headache free for days or weeks until the next attack. The severity of each migraine episode may vary.

MIGRAINE WARNING SIGNS

The best-known warning sign before a migraine is a migraine aura. In adults, auras are typically changes in the vision, such as zigzag lines, blind spots, shimmering lights, or colored balls. Auras occur in about 20 percent of people with migraine. Kids often have very elaborate auras, such as seeing things get bigger or smaller, like Alice in her Wonderland. Less commonly, people may experience numbness or weakness on one side of the body during a migraine aura.

Auras usually occur about thirty to sixty minutes before the painful part of the migraine and last for about five to twenty minutes. Although auras can be frightening when they first occur, they provide a unique opportunity to recognize a migraine early and treat it before painful symptoms begin. Most migraineurs who experience an aura also have migraine attacks that begin without an aura. Often these are milder. The migraine aura may occur without any headache, although this is more common in older migraineurs.

About 30 percent of migraine sufferers experience migraine prodromes (Kelman 2004). A *prodrome* is a warning that precedes the migraine by up to forty-eight hours. Unlike the very characteristic migraine auras, prodromes are often more vague. The most common prodromes include:

- fatigue
- mood change (either depression or euphoria)
- gastrointestinal symptoms (diarrhea, constipation, lack of interest in food)
- neck or head pain
- eye problems or vision changes
- sensitivity to light or noise
- dizziness
- difficulty concentrating
- food cravings

As with aura, recognizing prodromes can help you identify very early stages of migraine, when you can start treatment to prevent the painful stages of migraine.

MIGRAINE IS NOT AN EVERYDAY HEADACHE

Perhaps you believe that you have migraines every day. Actually, migraine is not a constant, continuous, or daily headache. Migraine is an intermittent, moderate or severe headache. A minority of people get migraines several days a week. This is *chronic migraine* and is treated with headache prevention therapies.

Some migraineurs, however, do have daily or very frequent headaches. When this happens, you have migraine

Exercise: Take the Migraine Quiz

Answer the following questions for your most severe headache. Answer the questions a second time if you also have a second, milder headache.

1. Does pain focus on one side of your head (left or right) at any point during the headache?

2. Does the pain feel like a pulsing, pounding, or throbbing?

3. Do you sometimes cut back on your activities when you have this headache?

4. Will the pain get worse if you walk up stairs or bend forward and put your head between your knees?

   Also answer the following three questions:

A. Do you try to turn down lights or close the blinds during this headache?

B. Do you try to reduce noise or seek quiet during this headache?

C. Do you feel nauseated or sometimes vomit with this headache?

   If you answered yes to at least two of the four numbered questions and one of the three lettered questions, your headache is probably a migraine. Remember that one of your headaches may be a migraine and another headache may have a different diagnosis. Review your headache information and the result of the migraine quiz with your doctor to help establish a positive migraine diagnosis.

plus another type of headache. It is important to recognize if you have other headaches besides migraine so you can find the best treatment for your particular headache combination.

Recognize Typical Features of Other Headaches

Migraineurs often experience additional, nonmigraine headaches. It's important for headache sufferers to know which of their headaches are migraine and which may be other types of headache. Getting the correct headache diagnosis is the first step toward finding an effective treatment. Share the results of these quizzes with your doctor.

MEDICATION OVERUSE HEADACHE

I used to get headaches only once a month. I still get a bad migraine with my menstrual period, but I also have a dull headache that's there every day. The daily headache seems to get better after I take a couple of pain pills, but then it comes back a few hours later. I've tried a few different migraine medicines, and nothing really helps. Now my doctor tells me the pain pills are causing the headache. How can this be?

Medication overuse is one of the most common reasons for migraineurs to have everyday headaches that never really get better. People with a long history of migraine headaches often notice their headaches become more frequent. As headaches become more frequent, people begin to use more and more painkillers. After using either over-the-counter or prescription painkillers three or more days per week for about six weeks, many people will develop *medication overuse* or *rebound* headaches. What this means is that the excessive and regular use of pain medications has led to an increased frequency of headaches. Medication overuse headaches are usually resistant to migraine therapy.

People with no previous history of headache will rarely develop headaches from using pain medication daily. So, for example, taking daily pain medication for arthritis won't lead to daily headaches unless you also have migraines. Medication overuse headache most typically occurs in migraineurs, although it may also develop in people with tension-type or post-trauma headaches.

Medication overuse headaches are very different from migraine and have the following characteristics:

- Headache occurs daily or almost every day.
- Pain is over both sides of the head.
- Pain is a dull pressure.
- Pain is bothersome but does not limit activities.
- Lights and noises aren't avoided during this headache.
- Nausea and vomiting do not occur during this headache.

Remember that medication overuse headaches typically occur in people who also have migraine. So you will still have some regular migraine attacks in addition to these milder, daily headaches.

Medication overuse headache is important for two reasons:

- Daily pain medication tends to make headaches more frequent.
- Headache treatment does *not* work in people also using daily pain medications.

Remember, regularly using a single pain medication or combination of pain medications three or more days per week is a common reason for having frequent headaches and poor success with a wide variety of migraine therapies.

How Can Painkillers Cause Pain?

Medication overuse headaches are similar to caffeine withdrawal symptoms. The heavy coffee drinker wakes like a bear: *I need my morning coffee.* She's irritable, shaky, and has a mild headache. After a cup of coffee, she feels better. A few hours later, the caffeine wears off and she's back at the coffeepot, taking another dose of caffeine. She knows she feels crummy every few hours due to caffeine withdrawal. If she stops drinking coffee altogether, she'll be miserable for a few weeks. Eventually, she'll no longer wake up each morning feeling cranky and headachy.

The same happens with painkillers in migraine sufferers. They wake up with a headache, take a couple of pain pills, and feel better for a few hours. Then the headache comes back, and they repeat their pain medication. If they don't take any pain pills for a few days or a couple of weeks, the headache may even get temporarily worse. After discontinuing all pain pills for two to four months, 65 to 85 percent of people who were previously overusing medications will find that their headaches are reduced by at least half (Rapoport et al. 1986). Overusing many medications designed to treat a migraine attack may result in medication overuse headache, including over-the-counter or prescription painkillers and other acute migraine therapies, like the triptans. (See chapter 4 for proper use of acute migraine medications.)

A more scientific explanation of medication overuse headache involves *down-regulation,* which is the brain's way of ignoring a message it hears over and over. Have you ever noticed how a new mother jumps every time her baby whimpers, while the seasoned mother can continue working despite a toddler screaming nearby? She has learned to tune out the everyday screaming fits. Every mother knows, though, when a "different" cry occurs that may signal a serious problem or injury and will immediately go on the alert when the cry changes.

The nerve cells in the brain use this same system. When they first see a pain pill, they block pain messages. When the nerve cells see pain pills day in and day out, they become accustomed to them and begin to ignore them. The more pain pills you take, the more the brain ignores them. Eventually, you may be taking excessive amounts of lots of different pills and notice the pain actually seems to be getting worse. This is because those pills are becoming less and less effective in the brain. Switching to a different brand or type of pain pill usually doesn't help, because all of these pills look the same to the

Exercise: Take the Medication Overuse Headache Quiz

This is the one quiz that you should answer by lumping all of your headaches together. Only answer these questions once.

1. Do you regularly have headaches four or more days per week?

2. Do you typically have four or more days per week when you need to take over-the-counter or prescription drugs for pain or headache? If you take a baby aspirin every day for heart disease, do not count that in your calculations.

If you answered yes to either of these questions, you are at risk for medication overuse headache. Some people with frequent headaches do not realize how much medication they actually are using. So if you have frequent headaches and don't think you overuse headache medications, keep a diary of all headache medication for one month to make sure (a diary is provided in chapter 3). Be sure to record both over-the-counter and prescription medications.

brain. Once you stop taking pain pills every day, it takes the brain several weeks to months to become interested in the messages sent with pain pills again. This is why it takes weeks to months for medication overuse headaches to improve after you discontinue daily pain pills.

Review this information with your doctor to decide if you're overusing medication. In general, you should have at least four days per week when you're not using a medication designed to treat a migraine episode, other headaches, or other pains. Appropriate treatment for frequent headache is described in chapter 5.

TENSION-TYPE HEADACHE

Three or four days each week, I get headaches that feel like a tight band pulled across my forehead. The headaches usually come on midday at work and last until I go to bed. The headaches don't limit my activities, but the nagging pain makes me feel depressed.

The main characteristic of tension-type headache is mild pain affecting both sides of the head. Unlike people with migraine, those with tension-type headache don't usually need to miss work or go lie down, and they are rarely nauseated. Tension-type headache tends to last longer than migraine, and some people seem to have the same headache for days, weeks, or even months.

Tension-type headaches used to be called "tension head-aches," "muscle contraction headaches," and "stress head-aches." The name was changed because the older names suggested false causes for the headaches. Muscle contraction or muscle tension occurs with both tension-type and migraine headache. In addition, stress is a trigger for most common headaches. "Tension-type" is also not a good name, but that is the current term being used.

Many doctors believe that tension-type headache is really a mild form of migraine. Most medications and nonmedication treatments work for both migraine and tension-type headaches. In addition, some people notice that a mild tension-type headache may develop into a migraine as the headache becomes more severe or if treatment doesn't work. Even though tension-type headache is milder than migraine, it is disruptive simply because these headaches can be so frequent.

Exercise: Take the Tension-Type Headache Quiz

Answer the following questions for your most severe headache. Answer the questions a second time if you also have a second, milder headache.

1. Is your pain usually on both sides of the head or across the forehead?

2. Does your pain feel like a pressure or squeezing?

3. Are you able to keep up with your usual routine despite your headache?

4. Can you walk up stairs and bend forward without your headache getting worse?

5. Are you still able to eat when you have a headache?

If you answered yes to at least three of these questions, your headache is probably a tension-type headache. Remember that you may have one headache that's a migraine and another that's a tension-type headache.

POST-TRAUMA HEADACHE

I never had headaches until my car accident, when I was rear-ended at a stop sign. Initially I was dazed and had severe neck and head pain. Over the next two weeks, I had an excruciating, constant headache and my family complained that I was irritable, moody, and forgetful. After a couple of weeks, my memory and mood improved. The headaches also became less constant. Six months later, I feel fine, except for intermittent, severe headaches once or twice a week.

Post-trauma headaches occur within two weeks of having a head injury with a concussion. Signs of a concussion include feeling dazed, seeing stars, being unable to remember what happened before or after the accident, or having lost consciousness. After a concussion, several other problems can arise:

- headache

- depressed or irritable mood

- memory loss

- dizziness or vertigo

- ringing in the ears

Headaches after a concussion may initially be severe and constant but usually become milder and less frequent after a couple of weeks. About 60 percent of people will continue to have post-trauma headaches for at least eight weeks (Lance and Arciniegas 2002). Headaches will continue for six to twelve months in only about one-third of people (Packard 1992). Headache characteristics may be similar to either migraine or tension-type headache, although tension-type symptoms are more common. Preexisting migraines may become more frequent after an accident. Post-trauma headaches are more likely to occur when your head was turned to the side and you were unaware of impending danger at the time of the accident.

Exercise: Take the Post-Trauma Headache Quiz

Answer the following questions for your most severe headache. Answer the questions a second time if you also have a second, milder headache.

1. Have you ever had a blow to the head that left you feeling dazed or stunned?

2. Have you ever had a head injury that knocked you out or left you unable to remember things that happened before or after the injury?

3. Did your headache begin within fourteen days of a head injury?

4. Did your headache pattern change within fourteen days of a head injury?

If you answered yes to question one or two, you probably had a concussion and are at risk for post-trauma headache. If you also answered yes to question three or four, you probably do have a post-trauma headache. If you have had a head injury and developed a headache afterward, that headache should get better over weeks to months. If your post-trauma headache is getting worse, see your doctor.

CLUSTER HEADACHE

Every spring and fall, like clockwork, I get excruciating headaches. I feel fine when I go to bed, but I wake up after ninety minutes with a horrific, unbearable pain in my left eye. I get out of bed and take a shower or start smoking and pacing around the room. Sometimes I bang my head against the wall or with a heavy book. After about an hour, the headache's totally gone and I go back to sleep, knowing that I'll wake up three more times for the same episode. Once these headaches start, I get them every night for the next six weeks. Then, as if by magic, they go away for several months. My wife gets migraines and always tries to get me to lie quietly with the headache. She'll often ask, "How bad can it be? The pain's gone in an hour." She's even beginning to wonder if I should see a psychiatrist.

Cluster headaches have the most distinctive features of all common headaches. They occur in groups or *clusters,* with headaches daily for several weeks, followed by months or even years with no headache. Cluster headaches usually occur at night, just when people begin to have dream sleep. During the day, these folks are often headache free.

Cluster headaches are very different from migraine. Each cluster headache episode is relatively brief, but the pain is much more intense than with migraine. People with recurring bouts of severe eye pain lasting thirty to ninety minutes may in fact have cluster headache. When medical books talk about cluster headaches, they focus on looking for a runny nose, tearing eyes, and decreased size of the pupil during the headache. People with cluster headaches rarely notice these changes because the pain is so intense. Behaviors during a cluster headache are also very different from migraine behaviors. Migraineurs can't stand movement, noise, or cigarette smoke. People with cluster headaches are the opposite: they avoid lying still, make noise, and sometimes smoke heavily during the headache. Cluster headache sufferers often engage in bizarre behaviors, like putting heavy pressure on the eye or temple, hitting the head, or firmly scratching a different part of the head. These behaviors may make both the cluster sufferer and his family wonder if he's "going crazy."

In the 1960s, cluster headache was a man's headache, with men affected six times as often as women. Today, men are only twice as likely to get cluster headache as women. Cluster headache has been linked to cigarette smoking. Some researchers think that increased smoking and other lifestyle changes in women may have contributed to the rising occurrence of cluster headache in women.

Exercise: Take the Cluster Headache Quiz

Answer the following questions for your most severe headache. Answer the questions a second time if you also have a second, milder headache.

1. Do you get an excruciating pain behind the eye?

2. Does this pain typically last three hours or less?

3. Do your headaches usually occur at night?

4. Do your headaches occur daily for several weeks, followed by months with none of these headaches?

If you answered yes to at least three of the questions above, you probably have cluster headache. Usually, people with cluster headache only have the one type of headache. Occasionally, migraineurs will also have cluster headaches.

Don't Be Fooled by Sinus Headache

Sinus headache generally occurs in association with a sinus infection or allergy symptoms. Migraineurs may incorrectly call their headaches "sinus headaches" because migraine pain is often located over the forehead and cheeks (where the sinuses are), because many seemingly sinus-related symptoms also occur during migraines, and because some sinus medications (like antihistamines) can effectively treat migraine.

Headache experts evaluated nearly 3,000 people with presumed sinus headache (Schreiber et al. 2004). Migraine was diagnosed in 80 percent of these patients. Most of the patients diagnosed with migraine had several sinus headache–like symptoms:

- sinus pressure (84 percent)

- sinus pain (82 percent)

- nasal congestion (63 percent)

- runny nose (40 percent)

- watery eyes (38 percent)

- itchy nose (27 percent)

In these patients, the frequent occurrence of pain around the area of the sinuses, nasal congestion and drainage, and tearing eyes had often led to the false conclusion that the migraine was a sinus headache. True sinus headaches typically occur in association with a sinus infection (when you would probably have a fever) or an allergy (when you also have tearing eyes, sneezing, and other allergy symptoms). Sinus pain is also generally relieved when the sinuses drain. If you think you have sinus headache, talk to your doctor to make sure you are not missing a migraine.

When It's More Than Just Migraine

My headaches just don't seem to fit into any one headache category. I've read about all the different kinds of headache, and I still don't know what I have.

Headache descriptions are always based on what is typical in the average headache sufferer. Your brain, however, doesn't really care what features are supposed to occur during a migraine, and you may have headache features that don't fit neatly into any one category. Every year, the National Headache Foundation sponsors a migraine art competition, where migraineurs submit artwork showing their headache attacks. These paintings commonly show a mixture of typical migraine features and typical tension-type headache features occurring in the same person. One artist painted a spike being hammered into one eye along with a clamp across both sides of the head. This shows the characteristic pounding pain of migraine, along with the pain on both sides of the head expected with tension-type headache. Headaches are diagnosed by the overall pattern of symptoms. You don't need to have only characteristics of migraine to be diagnosed with migraine headaches.

Sometimes, it can be hard to make a diagnosis because you have a couple of different types of headaches and have trouble remembering which headache had pain on one side of the head, which headache had sensitivity to light, and so on. In this case, tracking your headache symptoms using a diary (provided in chapter 3) can be very helpful.

Migraineurs often notice a change in their headaches over the years. This change has been called *transformed migraine*. The most common change is from infrequent, incapacitating migraines to milder headaches several days a week or every day. As mentioned in chapter 1, this change may reflect brain plasticity, or the brain learning to send pain messages more efficiently over time. This transformation usually occurs slowly. A gradual change from infrequent migraines to daily headaches may also be due to overuse of pain medications, development of new health problems, use of new medications (especially hormones), or a change in life stressors. An abrupt change in headache pattern may occur with head or neck trauma or new health problems. Migraineurs may also develop a second, distinct type of headache, like migraine plus tension-type headache. Cluster headaches are unusual in migraineurs. You should see your doctor any time there is a major change in your headache pattern.

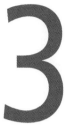

3

Track Your Symptoms and Triggers

When my doctor told me to keep a headache diary, I didn't think it would help. I've been living with these headaches for years. What good would it do to write things down? After a few weeks, though, the diary really surprised me by showing how often I actually have headaches and how they're often triggered by skipping meals and stress.

It's surprising how hard it can be to accurately remember headaches. People's recollection of pain is poor compared with their daily pain diaries (Stone et al. 2004). People often focus on their last or worst headache, forgetting about other attacks. It's also hard to remember what lifestyle changes or foods may have triggered a migraine on any given day.

Keep a Headache Diary

I thought I knew everything about my migraines, but keeping a diary showed me how my migraines start every week when I'm finishing up my weekly payroll. I also wasn't aware that sleeping in on the weekends was contributing to my migraines.

Keeping a headache diary for several weeks or months provides valuable information for you and your doctor. Diaries are effective tools to establish a headache diagnosis. They frequently show that headache pattern and frequency are different from a person's memory of the migraine. For example, what were assumed to be menstrual migraines may actually be occurring throughout the month and not just with menses. Diaries may also identify a pattern of medication overuse or reveal previously undetected migraine triggers. After you keep a headache diary for several weeks, you may want to retake the quizzes in chapter 2 to see if your answers have changed.

Diaries can also reveal typical headache patterns. For example, your headache may begin with a prodrome of irritability and chocolate craving six hours before the headache. Your headaches may frequently occur four hours after a stressful day at work or when you've skipped lunch. Identifying these patterns can help you predict when a migraine might occur so you can use migraine therapies early, before a painful headache begins. For example, you might take your usual migraine pill during a prodrome or plan a relaxing walk or stretching exercises when you've completed a stressful workday.

Migraine patterns and prodromes can be different for different people. This means you have to play detective and look for the pattern that occurs with your headaches. Tracking symptoms is the best way to piece together clues to establish your own pattern.

Daily Headache Diary						
Date: _____						
Time of Day	Severity					Medications
	1	2	3	4	5	
Morning						
Noon						
Evening						
Bedtime						
List nonmedication treatment strategies used:						

Migraine Symptoms

☐ one-sided pain

☐ throbbing or pulsing

☐ decreased activities

☐ reduced lights

☐ reduced noises

☐ avoided smells

☐ felt nauseated or vomited

Prodrome and Aura

- ☐ fatigue
- ☐ mood change
- ☐ digestive or stomach problem
- ☐ neck or head pain
- ☐ eye problem or vision change
- ☐ sensitivity to lights or noise
- ☐ dizziness
- ☐ difficulty concentrating
- ☐ food craving
- ☐ aura
- ☐ _____
- ☐ _____

Triggers

- ☐ menses
- ☐ stress
- ☐ glare
- ☐ skipped a meal
- ☐ too much sleep
- ☐ too little sleep
- ☐ odor
- ☐ change in weather
- ☐ exercise
- ☐ alcohol
- ☐ caffeine
- ☐ chocolate
- ☐ tomatoes, tomato sauce
- ☐ peanut butter
- ☐ processed meats
- ☐ canned food
- ☐ Chinese food
- ☐ aspartame
- ☐ broad beans
- ☐ _____
- ☐ _____

Using the Headache Diary

Complete this headache diary every day for four to eight weeks. It often takes several weeks or even a couple of months to identify headache patterns, especially if you have fairly infrequent headaches. Fill in the diary daily, whether you have a headache or not, so you can look for differences in triggers or prodromal symptoms on days with and without headaches. Record every headache, not just the most severe ones.

By discovering your own headache pattern, you can decide:

- if mild headaches will probably turn into migraines

- when nonmedication remedies are likely to be helpful

- when medications are most likely to work

Record your headache severity four times daily. Migraine symptoms, prodrome and aura, and triggers should be recorded once daily. If you identify prodromes, auras, or triggers not included on this list, write them in the blanks.

MEASURE HEADACHE SEVERITY

Log your headache severity using this scale:

0 = no headache

1 = you feel pain only if you think about it

2 = mild pain that can be ignored

3 = moderate pain that reduces productivity or efficiency

4 = severe pain that limits your activities

5 = incapacitating headache that prevents all activities

Recording headaches four times daily helps to show how severe your headache is and how long it lasts. With treatment, you may notice a reduction in the headache severity or the length of your migraine episodes. Improvement in either maximum severity or migraine duration means that your treatment is beginning to work.

RECORD MEDICATIONS

Before keeping a diary, I had no idea how much medicine I was using. Both my doctor and I became concerned about what all those painkillers could be doing to my health.

In addition to having poor memory for pain, people tend to underestimate the amount of medications they use. The diary can help you keep track of how much medication you are using. Log every medication you use to treat migraine or pain. Other drugs can have an effect on migraines, so record any medications you use infrequently to see if they're triggering your headaches. You don't need to record non-pain medications that you take the same way every day.

Record both over-the-counter and prescription medications. This is especially important to make sure you haven't developed medication overuse headaches. Taking any pain pill—over-the-counter or prescription—three or more days each week puts you at risk. If you take aspirin twice a week, acetaminophen twice a week, and a prescription migraine pill twice a week, you may think you're okay because no medication is used more than twice a week. However, all pain pills break down into similar compounds in the body, so switching between pain remedies won't reduce your risk of medication overuse headache. Your goal is to have at least four days each week when you don't use any pain medicines. However, having a couple of bad weeks in a row won't worsen headaches. It usually takes about six weeks of regular pain medication use to develop medication overuse headache.

The medication log can also be used to see how medications work best for you. You may notice, for example, that your migraine therapy works well if you take it when the pain is at a severity of three, but not if you wait until it reaches four or five. Your medication may work best if you take it during a prodrome or aura, before migraine pain begins.

MONITOR MIGRAINE SYMPTOMS

Tracking migraine symptoms can help you identify which of your headaches are migraines. You may notice that a mild headache still has several migraine features. This headache may be a migraine, even though it's not severe. Most migraineurs have a mixture of moderate and severe migraines.

MONITOR PRODROME SYMPTOMS

Prodrome symptoms usually occur within about six hours of the onset of a migraine. In some people, prodrome symptoms precede the migraine by up to two days. When you have a migraine, it's hard to remember what happened hours earlier. Keep track of possible prodromes every day, whether you have a headache or not. This way, you can look back at the diaries to notice trends. For example, you may discover that you typically crave chocolate the night before a migraine, or morning fatigue may predict an afternoon headache. If you can identify prodromes, you can use either migraine medications or nonmedication therapy during a prodrome to help prevent the painful part of the migraine.

MONITOR POSSIBLE TRIGGERS

Monitoring the effects of common migraine triggers on your headaches can help reveal which factors may be triggers for you. If you can identify triggers, you can:

- reduce exposure to some triggers (like excessive sleep or skipping meals)
- change your reaction to triggers you can't avoid (like stress)
- start preventive strategies when you're exposed to a trigger

You may find that your migraines occur after you're exposed to a combination of triggers, such as stress plus skipping a meal. Not everyone will be able to identify triggers.

Most triggers should provoke a migraine within about twelve hours. So work stress, skipping lunch, or drinking four cups of coffee on Monday cannot be blamed for Wednesday's migraine. In addition, most triggers will not always produce a headache. For many people, the amount of exposure to a single trigger matters. In others, the additive effects of trigger combinations are necessary to provoke migraines.

One can of diet soda is okay for me, but if I drink several cans or eat lots of diet foods containing aspartame, I'll get a migraine for sure.

Usually, I can eat whatever I want. But if I overdo it on coffee on a high-stress day, watch out! I'll almost always get a migraine then.

When my period's going to start, I know I need to get regular sleep and not skip breakfast like I usually do. Otherwise, I'll get a terrible migraine.

Analyzing Your Diary

Evaluating your particular headache pattern helps you identify:

- the type of headache you have
- when your headache is becoming a migraine
- when you should start migraine treatment

- what factors predict your migraine

If you have headaches every day or many days a week, you may not be able to link prodrome symptoms or triggers to your headaches.

FINDING A HEADACHE PATTERN

Different headaches will have different patterns. Usually, migraineurs will have no headache recorded on most days, with occasional episodes of moderate to severe pain (severity of three to five) lasting for several hours. Tension-type headache will be mild (severity of one to three) and may last for several days. Cluster headache would be a short headache, at bedtime only, probably recorded as a severity of five and typically occurring every night for several weeks.

You may also notice that you have a mild daily headache (severity of one to two) and a moderate to severe headache (severity of three to four) once or twice a week. This pattern often represents the combination of migraine and tension-type headache. A similar pattern is also seen with migraine plus medication overuse headaches. If you do have migraine and tension-type headaches, it is important to recognize when a headache is turning into a migraine, so you can treat it early to prevent a disabling migraine. Some people notice, for example, that once a headache reaches a severity of three, it usually becomes a migraine.

IF YOU HAVE HEADACHES FEWER THAN THREE DAYS PER WEEK

Headaches are easiest to analyze when you have no headache most days of the week. If your headaches occur twice a week or less often, look at those prodrome factors and triggers that occurred on the day of your headache and also the day before your headache. If you find you're feeling fatigue or craving sweets on most days, whether you get a headache or not, these are not prodromes for you. True prodromes are present before at least half of your headaches. Answer these questions about prodromes you believe predict your migraine:

- Did the prodrome occur before at least half of your migraines?

- When the prodrome occurred, did a migraine follow at least half the time?

If you can answer yes to both of these questions, you have found a reliable prodrome to predict your migraines.

Similarly, triggers usually produce headaches within twelve hours of exposure. So if you eat chocolate and hot dogs (processed meat) on Monday and don't have a headache until Wednesday, these foods were not triggers for that headache. As with prodromes, not every trigger will always lead to a headache. In many cases, triggers provoke a headache only when you are already predisposed to one. Many people find that it takes a combination of triggers to tip the scale. For example, weekend headaches are thought to be provoked by the combination of sleeping in and missing breakfast. If you think you have identified a migraine trigger, answer these questions:

- Did a migraine occur within twelve hours after you were exposed to the trigger?

- Look at all the days when you were exposed to that trigger. Did a migraine occur at least half the time?

If you answered yes to both questions, you have successfully identified a migraine trigger.

Try to link migraine prodromes and triggers. In some cases, a possible trigger may actually be a reaction to the prodrome. For example, before a migraine, do you have food cravings (a prodrome) and eat some chocolate (a possible trigger)? Do you have diarrhea or constipation (a prodrome) and skip meals (a trigger) before a migraine? Or do you experience irritability (a prodrome) and react by feeling more stress at work (a trigger)? If you recognize these patterns, you can identify the prodrome, avoid exposing yourself to the trigger, and start preventive therapy. You might realize, *I'm really irritable, just got my menstrual period, and would kill for a chocolate–peanut butter bar! You know, I often feel like this a few hours before my migraine starts. I'll use this time to do some relaxation and stretching exercises to see if I can prevent this migraine from developing.* Research shows that taking migraine medication during a prodrome can effectively prevent the development of a migraine or reduce the severity of a migraine that does develop (Luciani et al. 2000).

IF YOU HAVE HEADACHES MORE THAN THREE DAYS PER WEEK

When you regularly have headaches three or more days each week, it is very difficult to identify prodromes and triggers. The exception is when you have frequent, very mild headaches with infrequent, severe migraines. In this case, you can sometimes identify prodromes and triggers occurring in advance of the severe headache. Even if you have frequent headaches, a diary can be useful in helping you recognize types of headache and monitoring medication use. Diaries can also be used to compare headaches before and after treatment.

HOW TO TELL IF YOUR HEADACHES ARE IMPROVING

A few lucky people notice dramatic improvement in their headaches with treatment. Most people, however, find that improvement occurs gradually. Sometimes, people stop a treatment that would eventually have been very effective because they didn't realize their headaches were starting to get better.

Use headache diaries to monitor your response to treatment. Compare your notes over about four weeks. Answer these questions:

- Are you having fewer episodes of severe headache?

- Do you have more days that are free from any headache?

- Are your headache severity scores generally lower?

- Are you experiencing fewer migraine symptoms with your headaches?

If you answered yes to any of these questions, your headaches are probably improving. Save your diaries so you can look for long-term changes.

When Should You Use a Headache Diary?

Completing daily diaries takes time, and you don't need to keep diaries forever. Diaries are most useful to:

- identify a headache diagnosis

- discover patterns of frequency and severity

- evaluate response to a new therapy

Migraine therapies include acute treatments (those designed to treat an individual headache episode) and preventive treatments (those designed to reduce future headache severity and frequency). When trying a new acute migraine treatment, keep a daily diary until you have used the new treatment for at least three headaches. When starting a new preventive treatment, record daily headache activity for at least three months. Keep additional diaries to monitor your response when your treatment is adjusted.

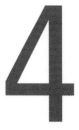

Treat Acute Migraine Symptoms

I'm not sure how to use my pills. First my doctor told me I was using my migraine pill too often. Then he gave me a new pill and told me to take it every day. Why are the directions different this time?

Migraine medications can be divided into acute and preventive therapies. Acute therapies are used to treat a specific migraine episode. If used too frequently, acute therapies can cause medication overuse headache. Preventive therapy, as you might guess, is designed to prevent future headaches. Preventive therapies must be used every day to work and take about two to three months to start working. Preventive medications will not help the headache you have today, tomorrow, or even next week. Preventive therapy is designed to reduce long-term headache frequency and severity.

Acute medication:	Preventive medication:
• treats today's migraine	• prevents future migraines
• is used for infrequent or severe migraines	• is used for frequent headaches
• should be taken no more than three days per week	• must be used every day

People with frequent headaches often use a daily preventive therapy, plus acute therapy when they have a severe migraine. It is essential to know which of your medications is designed to treat the headache you have today and which is used to prevent future headaches. This chapter will discuss effective acute medication. Migraine prevention medications will be discussed in the next chapter.

How Do You Know If Your Acute Medication Is Working?

Migraineurs often settle for poor headache relief, thinking that any relief is better than no relief. To see if your acute migraine medication is doing its job, take the acute migraine medication quiz.

WHY DON'T YOUR ACUTE MIGRAINE MEDICATIONS WORK BETTER?

Different medications work for different people. Even if your mother gets relief from one medication, you may need a different therapy. Let your doctor know if you're not getting good relief from your medicine. Doctors have not been trained to ask patients how well a medication works. Doctors will ask, "Is this medication helpful?" However, the doctor really wants to know how effectively the migraine is eliminated, how fast

Exercise: Acute Migraine Medication Quiz

1. Two hours after taking your acute migraine medication, do you still have substantial pain, sensitivity to light and sound, or nausea?

2. Do you usually need to take two or more doses before the pain goes away?

3. Do you use some acute migraine medication three or more days every week?

4. Do you use over-the-counter painkillers for your headache almost every day?

5. Do you or your friends, family, or doctors worry that you're overusing your migraine medication?

If you answered yes to any of these questions, you are probably not achieving optimal relief from your current migraine medications.

the medicine works, and whether you have side effects. Use the satisfaction assessment provided later in this chapter to answer these important questions.

Regular use of acute migraine medications must be limited to no more than a couple of days per week. If you usually use some acute medication three or more days per week, you are at risk for developing medication overuse headache. Acute migraine medications will not effectively relieve migraines when medications are being overused. If you think you might be overusing acute medications, keep track of your medication use and review it with your doctor.

How Should You Use Acute Migraine Medications?

Acute migraine medications work best if used early in a migraine episode. In general, acute treatment will relieve your migraine most effectively if you take the medication when symptoms are still mild to moderate. Studies also show that migraine medicines work best when taken before the nerves become sensitized (Burstein, Collins, and Jakubowski 2004). You can identify when your nerves have become sensitized because you will develop allodynia, or an increased sensitivity of the skin to touch. Most people feel this as a tender scalp or feeling like the head is swollen. So pay attention to how long it takes for your hair to hurt or for your glasses or earrings to feel uncomfortably tight during a migraine. You should take your acute medications before these changes occur.

Use a medication to treat at least three separate migraines before deciding whether it's working for you. Record each episode in your diary (see chapter 3) so you can determine whether the medication helped, how long it took for your migraine to get better, and any patterns that suggest you might be able to take it earlier next time. Often, people delay migraine treatment with a new medication until the symptoms are severe.

I'm kind of afraid to try new pills. But my migraine is so bad now, I don't care what side effects the pill causes. Nothing could be as bad as this migraine! These pills are really expensive, so I try to save them until the pain is unbearable and nothing else has helped.

Delaying treatment usually reduces the degree of migraine relief. Once people get some relief from a new pill, they feel more comfortable treating their next migraine and will treat earlier, milder symptoms. They often notice their relief is much better with the second migraine than the first. Also, once in a while you will get a killer migraine that acute medication really doesn't help. If that's the only migraine you treat with a new remedy, you may abandon a treatment that could have worked well for your more typical attacks.

Effective Over-the-Counter Medications

Every TV advertisement for pain medicine claims that four out of five doctors recommend this pill as the best headache remedy. What I want to know is, have these doctors ever tried these pills themselves? They sure don't work for me!

A survey of over 8,000 migraineurs in England and the United States showed that 52 percent used only over-the-counter medications to treat their headaches (Lipton et al. 2003). Another 23 percent of migraineurs used both over-the-counter and prescription medications. In both countries, the most commonly used over-the-counter medication was acetaminophen (Tylenol), followed by ibuprofen (Motrin, Advil) and then caffeine/aspirin/acetaminophen combination products (like Excedrin). Unfortunately, this survey also showed that 75 percent of migraineurs in both countries still had substantial disability with their migraines, suggesting poor benefit from their treatments.

Not all over-the-counter treatments are equally effective. Also, treatment response usually varies depending on how severe a migraine is when it's treated. Fortunately, a lot of good research has provided a basis for good recommendations about which over-the-counter medications work the best and how to use them most effectively.

ASPIRIN, ACETAMINOPHEN, OR IBUPROFEN?

Drugstore displays proudly announce that acetaminophen is the number one headache remedy. The study by Lipton and colleagues (2003) does show that acetaminophen is the most *frequently used* over-the-counter migraine treatment. Interestingly, although acetaminophen is one of the most effective medications for other pain, like arthritis, it is probably the least effective over-the-counter acute migraine treatment.

Aspirin, acetaminophen, and ibuprofen may all reduce migraine severity. Aspirin alone is actually as effective as acetaminophen combined with codeine (Boureau et al. 1994). In addition, nonsteroidal anti-inflammatory medications, such as naproxen (Aleve) or ibuprofen, usually provide better migraine relief than acetaminophen. Ibuprofen and naproxen are also more effective for treating tension-type headache than acetaminophen (Miller et al. 1987; Schachtel, Furey, and Thoden 1996).

Although aspirin, ibuprofen, and naproxen are more effective in relieving headaches, they can have troublesome side effects. Common side effects include stomach upset, bleeding, and dizziness. Many people use acetaminophen because they tolerate it better than aspirin, ibuprofen, or naproxen. People with a history of bleeding problems or stomach ulcers generally use acetaminophen.

ADDING CAFFEINE IMPROVES RELIEF

My doctor told me to cut out caffeine to help my migraines. Then he told me to take a painkiller that has caffeine in it. What's up with that?

Interestingly, although caffeine withdrawal is a common trigger for migraineurs who drink more than two cups of coffee a day, caffeine is frequently included in acute migraine medications. In addition to acting as a stimulant, caffeine actually increases the effect of *analgesic* (painkilling) medications. About 40 to 60 percent of people will have migraine relief with over-the-counter analgesics (Boureau et al. 1994; Miller et al. 1987; Schachtel, Furey, and Thoden 1996). This relief can be improved by adding caffeine to the analgesic. For example, adding 100 milligrams of caffeine to a nonsteroidal anti-inflammatory medication increased the number of people who got migraine relief by one and one-half times (Peroutka et al. 2004). Caffeine is often included in over-the-counter analgesics, like Excedrin (65 milligrams caffeine per tablet) and Anacin (32 milligrams caffeine per tablet).

If you don't have an analgesic plus caffeine medication at home, you can add caffeine yourself by taking your over-the-counter analgesic with a caffeinated beverage. Amounts of caffeine in common beverages are:

coffee (7 ounces)	65–135 milligrams caffeine
tea (7 ounces)	40–60 milligrams caffeine
cola (12 ounces)	30–50 milligrams caffeine

Most people don't get caffeine withdrawal headache unless they are regularly consuming the equivalent of about two cups of coffee daily. Avoid caffeinated medications if you are especially sensitive to caffeine or your doctor has asked you to eliminate caffeine.

DO OVER-THE-COUNTER MEDICATIONS REALLY WORK?

The combination of an analgesic with caffeine probably gives the best over-the-counter pain relief. Both Excedrin and Anacin offer this combination. Excedrin has been scientifically evaluated in several large, national research studies. These studies have generally shown that Excedrin relieves migraine in about 60 percent of migraineurs. These studies, however, excluded people with severe migraines, including those who would go to bed with their headaches or would occasionally vomit with their migraines.

HOW SHOULD YOU USE OVER-THE-COUNTER MEDICATIONS?

Over-the-counter medications can be effective for migraines that are mild or moderately severe. Treating the headache early, while it is still mild, should improve your migraine relief. Use your diary to find out which over-the-counter medications work best for you and how early you need to take them to get good relief. As with all acute migraine therapies, don't use over-the-counter medications more than three days per week.

Here are guidelines for effective use of over-the-counter medications:

- Aspirin, ibuprofen, and naproxen are generally more effective than acetaminophen.

- Use acetaminophen if you don't tolerate the other analgesics.

- Use acetaminophen if you have a bleeding disorder or gastric ulcers.

- Add caffeine to analgesics to improve pain relief.

- Limit over-the-counter drugs to three or fewer days per week.

- Let your doctor know about your over-the-counter drug use.

Remind your doctor about any over-the-counter medications you use. Sometimes, your doctor may not want you to use a particular medication because it will interact with another therapy or worsen another health condition.

Always follow the directions on the labels of over-the-counter medications. Usually, you won't get any better relief by taking an excessively high dose of over-the-counter medication. For example, for most people, taking 800 milligrams of ibuprofen doesn't work any better for reducing pain than taking 400 milligrams. Even though the pain relief will be the same, you'll probably have more side effects with a higher dosage. If you have long-lasting headaches, taking a lower dose more often generally works better than taking a high dose less often. For example, acetaminophen is usually taken every four to six hours. If your dose doesn't work when you take it every six hours, try taking the same dose every four hours rather than increasing the dose you take every six hours. Taking a lower dose more frequently helps maintain an effective drug level in your system. Taking a high dose infrequently causes high and low levels of the drug throughout the day, with an effective level achieved for just a short time.

Effective Prescription Migraine Drugs

Prescription acute migraine medications include medications designed to relieve nausea, sedatives, and the migraine-specific drugs DHE and the triptans. Among these categories, the migraine-specific drugs are the most effective acute migraine medications.

ANTINAUSEA MEDICATIONS

Medications designed to reduce nausea, like prochlorperazine (Compazine), often reduce other migraine symptoms. Antinausea medications can reduce both pain and nausea in migraineurs who have moderate to severe nausea with their migraines. Unfortunately, pain relief is usually short-lived if antinausea drugs are used without another migraine treatment.

Therefore, antinausea medications are best used in combination with an analgesic or a migraine-specific treatment (DHE or triptan). Many antinausea medications are available as rectal suppositories, which can be very helpful if severe nausea prevents you from taking oral medications.

SEDATIVES

Twenty years ago, sedatives were the mainstay of migraine therapy. Sleep helps to shut off the serotonin pain pathway. Also, if you sleep long enough, you may sleep through much of the painful part of the migraine. This is why, years ago, migraineurs with a severe attack were brought into the hospital and treated with sedatives so they would have a prolonged sleep. The development of more effective treatments eliminated this need to sleep away migraine days.

Some people still use sedatives for migraine, usually butalbital drugs (such as Fiorinal and Fioricet) and isometheptene mucate (Midrin). In these drugs, a sedative is combined with either aspirin or acetaminophen. Because the only painkiller in these drugs is aspirin or acetaminophen, they are not strong painkillers. Sedatives are sometimes helpful for people who know that their migraine will go away if they can sleep for thirty to sixty minutes. If they use a dose of medication to help them get to sleep, they may wake with good migraine relief.

Butalbital is a barbiturate, and it is habit-forming. If you begin using butalbital frequently, you can develop a dependency on it and find that you want to keep taking more. Butalbital is rarely effective for most migraineurs.

MIGRAINE-SPECIFIC TREATMENTS: DHE AND TRIPTANS

The medications discussed so far are all designed to treat other conditions besides migraine. The *ergotamines* and the *triptans* are two groups of medications that were specifically developed to treat migraine. These medications relieve migraine better than the over-the-counter analgesics.

Ergotamines

Ergotamines have been used to treat migraines for decades. Many older ergotamines, like Cafergot (ergotamine tartrate with caffeine), cause increased nausea, which limits their use. A newer ergotamine, dihydroergotamine or DHE, causes much less nausea. DHE may be administered as an injection with an antinausea medication for severe and long-lasting migraine attacks. DHE also comes in the form of a nasal spray (Migranal). DHE takes several hours to begin working, but the effects can last for days. For this reason, DHE nasal spray is often used by migraineurs whose attacks typically last longer than one day.

Triptans

The triptans are the other group of migraine-specific acute drugs. Triptans were designed to relieve migraine pain, nausea, and sensitivity to noise and lights. Like DHE, the triptans are very effective in relieving migraine. Unlike DHE, triptans provide rapid relief and have few limiting side effects.

There are several triptans available in a variety of dosage formulations. The fastest and most complete relief occurs with injectable sumatriptan (Imitrex). Nasal triptans also provide faster relief than pills, although they don't provide any better relief. Most patients prefer pills. Some triptans are available in a form that dissolves in the mouth without water. Both types of tablets work equally well.

A study of migraine patients at a specialty headache clinic found that only 19 percent failed to respond to at least one of three triptans (Mathew et al. 2000). So if you don't get relief after treating three migraines with one triptan, talk to your doctor about trying another triptan. If relief from the triptan doesn't last long enough, try taking an over-the-counter analgesic with the triptan. This may prolong headache relief (Krymchantowski and Barbosa 2002).

Migraine-Specific Treatments		
	Brand Name	**Effective Formulations**
Ergotamines		
dihydroergotamine	Migranal	1 milligram injection nasal spray
Triptans		
almotriptan	Axert	12.5 milligram tablet
eletriptan	Relpax	40 milligram tablet
frovatriptan	Frova	2.5 milligram tablet
naratriptan	Amerge	2.5 milligram tablet
rizatriptan	Maxalt	10 milligram dissolving tablet (MLT) 10 milligram tablet
sumatriptan	Imitrex	6 milligram injection nasal spray 50–100 milligram tablet
zolmitriptan	Zomig	nasal spray 5 milligram dissolving tablet (ZMT) 5 milligram tablet

If the first dose of DHE or a triptan is ineffective, it can be repeated after two hours, except for naratriptan, which can be repeated after four hours.

Both ergotamines and triptans can cause a small constriction in the blood vessels surrounding the heart. For this reason, these medications are usually not prescribed for people with heart disease, uncontrolled high blood pressure, or a history of strokes. Good health habits, like controlling blood pressure, lowering cholesterol, discontinuing nicotine use, and reducing obesity, can reduce risk for heart disease and stroke and make patients eligible to use some migraine-specific acute therapies.

RESCUE THERAPY

Rescue therapy is used when your usual acute treatment does not relieve your migraine symptoms. If you still have a headache several hours after using your triptan, you may take an analgesic such as aspirin, ibuprofen, or naproxen or a narcotic painkiller such as Vicodin (hydrocodone) or Percocet (oxycodone) as a rescue therapy. It's important to remember that narcotics are not very effective for migraines. For this reason, narcotics are not used as first-line or routine acute migraine therapy. If you find that you frequently need to take rescue medication because you're not getting adequate relief from your acute migraine medication, talk to your doctor about changing your acute therapy.

Which Treatment Should You Use?

Treatment selection will depend on your headache severity and symptoms. Here are some guidelines:

- Use analgesics when your migraine is mild with little disability.

- A caffeine-containing analgesic will probably work best.

- Consider adding an antinausea medication if needed.

- Use DHE or a triptan for severe or disabling migraines.

- Consider a different acute medication when you get poor relief or you usually need to repeat your dose for the same headache.

- Consider adding a preventive therapy if you usually need to use acute medication more than two days per week (see chapter 5).

Talk to your doctor to determine which acute treatment is right for you. Headache characteristics and other health problems may limit appropriate medication choices. Never use a medication that has been prescribed for someone else.

What Should You Expect from Acute Medication?

Target goals for acute medication typically include:

- relief of migraine symptoms within two hours

- no return of headache for at least twenty-four hours

- no side effects that make you reluctant to use your medication

While some people never achieve this level of relief with any treatment, these target goals can help you decide if you have been settling for an inadequate response. Failure to achieve a good treatment response should prompt you to consider a different treatment. Whenever your doctor gives you a new acute migraine medication, use these target goals to assess whether you're getting a good response.

Exercise: Take the Acute Migraine
Therapy Satisfaction Assessment

Try your acute migraine therapy for three
migraine episodes to accurately assess its effectiveness. Keep track of how well your treatment goals were met by answering these
questions for each of the three episodes. Write
down how long it took to achieve headache
relief. Circle yes or no for the remaining questions. Review your responses at your next
doctor's appointment.

Medication used: _____

Date: _____

1. How long did your migraine last after
   treatment? _____

2. Did you get relief fast enough?   Yes No

3. Did your migraine go away completely?
   Yes No

4. Were there side effects that make you
   hesitant to use this medication? Yes No

5. Are you satisfied with this treatment?
   Yes No

Enhance Migraine Relief with Neck Exercises

The following exercises can help minimize pain during a
migraine attack. These exercises can be used alone or in

combination with acute migraine medication. Apply heat or ice (whichever you find more soothing) for fifteen minutes to the neck and shoulders before and after these exercises.

OSCILLATORY MOVEMENTS. Sit up straight with your head facing forward. You will be repeatedly turning your chin toward one shoulder and back to the starting position. Make small, rhythmic movements, only moving your chin about two inches from the starting position and then back to straight ahead. First, turn your head away from the painful side and back. Repeat once per second for thirty seconds. Rest for thirty seconds. Repeat until no further relief is noted. Now switch to turning the head toward the painful side, and proceed as above.

POSITIONAL DISTRACTION. Place a one- to two-inch stack of books on the floor. Lie down with the back of your head resting on the books. The edge of the books should be near the middle of your head, so that your neck is free. Relax so that your head moves up from your neck.

TRIGGER POINT COMPRESSION. During a migraine, you may notice that pressure in certain places aggravates your head pain. These tender muscle spots are called *trigger points*. The shoulder and neck muscles often have trigger points that send pain into the side of your head. If you identify trigger points, apply pressure to them with your fingers and hold for twelve to sixty seconds. (While pressure may initially increase your pain, it causes a temporary decrease in blood flow to the painful area. When you let go, there is a surge of returning blood flow. Therapists think this helps wash away some of the chemicals that cause muscle tenderness and spasm.) Release the pressure, then proceed with the preventive stretching exercises introduced in chapter 5.

Acute Migraine Treatment in Women

Migraines occurring with the menstrual period are often more severe than nonmenstrual attacks. For this reason, many women need to use a migraine-specific treatment for menstrual migraines. Using an analgesic or triptan medication in low doses for five to six days around the menstrual period can reliably prevent severe headaches from occurring at this time. Specific regimens are discussed in the "Preventing Migraine in Women" section of chapter 5.

Acute migraine medication options are limited during pregnancy because of risks to the developing baby. Throughout pregnancy, acetaminophen may be safely used. Use of other analgesics is limited to the second trimester. Narcotic medications are sometimes used for infrequent, severe migraines. You should not use ergotamines when you're pregnant. The safety of triptans for the developing baby has not been tested. Registries of pregnant women who have inadvertently used triptans have not identified any specific birth defects, but too few babies have been evaluated to ensure that triptans are safe for the baby. Some doctors allow women to use injectable sumatriptan when nursing, since only minimal amounts of the drug are seen in the breast milk after an injection (Wojnar-Horton et al. 1996). Some doctors suggest pumping and discarding milk for four hours after using sumatriptan and using stored milk for feedings during that time. Any medication you are considering using while pregnant or breastfeeding should be reviewed in advance with your obstetrician and the baby's pediatrician.

Acute Migraine Treatment in Kids

Although you may want to give your kid a break when he has a migraine and keep him out of school for the day, this is usually not necessary unless he is vomiting or truly can't get to school. Migraines will probably last throughout the school years and may occur frequently. Missing school for migraine can result in excessive absences, which can harm school performance. Perhaps even more importantly, kids who miss school for migraine soon become isolated from their friends and peer groups. Teachers and peers often believe that the child is making up a headache complaint to avoid schoolwork. They may even resent these frequent absences, saying things like, "Boy, I'd like to stay home and watch TV every time I had a little headache."

So what should you do if your child gets migraines? First, see a doctor to get a diagnosis. Once you know the headache is not a sign of a more serious illness, you can:

- Send your child with migraine to school unless she is vomiting.

- Keep your child home if she is too sick for school in the morning; then take her once she feels better.

- Alert the school nurse to the headache diagnosis.

- Have acute medications available for the school nurse to administer.

Your child will have her migraine whether she's at home or at school. Attending school should not make the migraine worse. Most migraines in kids are short. Even if she has a headache in the morning, it will probably be gone in one to three hours. So it's better to give her medication and have her attend school. Also, pay attention to what symptoms occur before the bad migraine pain. Your child may notice that she typically feels dizzy, gets queasy, or starts yawning before a migraine. If she can identify migraine prodromes, she can treat her migraine before the pain begins.

The same principles for treating migraine in adults apply to children and adolescents. Although both ibuprofen and acetaminophen are used to treat migraines in kids, ibuprofen is twice as likely as acetaminophen to completely relieve a migraine within two hours (Hamalainen et al. 1997). The benefit of caffeine may be added by having children take ibuprofen with a half can of cola. In addition, isometheptene mucate (Midrin) is often more effective in children than adults. None of the triptans has been approved for use in children and adolescents. Several research studies, however, do show that children can safely use triptans for migraine (Lewis et al. 2004). The dosage needs to be adjusted for children, though, so they should never use adults' triptan prescriptions.

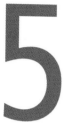

5

Use Medication and Nonmedication Therapies to Prevent Migraine

My doctor said my migraines aren't bad enough for migraine prevention. Even when I take medication, I still lose half a day with each attack. I've stopped going out in the evenings and traveling because of my migraines. How bad do they have to be before I can try to prevent them?

Migraine prevention is used daily over the long term to reduce the frequency and severity of migraine attacks. Unlike acute migraine therapy, migraine prevention does not treat a migraine you are having today. Obviously, everyone with migraines wants to prevent future migraines. Most people, however, don't want to take a migraine prevention drug or use nonmedication prevention every day unless their attacks are frequent or very disabling. For this reason, doctors usually don't discuss migraine prevention unless headaches usually occur several days per week.

How Do You Know If You Need Migraine Prevention?

Migraine prevention is typically used by people with:

- frequent migraines
- prolonged or disabling migraines
- migraines that respond poorly to acute therapy

If you usually have headaches three or more days per week, you are a candidate for prevention therapies. Migraine

---

Exercise: Take the Migraine Prevention Quiz

1. Do you usually have a migraine or other headache more than two days per week?

2. Even though you use an acute migraine therapy, do you miss school, work, or family activities at least once a week because of your migraine?

3. Do you overuse acute migraine medications to prevent a migraine from occurring?

If you answered yes to any of these questions, you should talk to your doctor about migraine prevention.

---

prevention may also be considered if acute medications are ineffective for you or you still have significant disability despite using acute medications. To see if you might be a candidate for migraine prevention, take this quiz.

How Should You Use Migraine Prevention?

Preventive therapies must be used every day to work. Most migraine prevention treatments won't improve your migraines until you have used them regularly for about two to three months. If your doctor prescribes a prevention medication and you forget to take it several days in a row, it will take even longer to achieve migraine relief. So if you can't remember to take preventive medications consistently, they probably won't work for you. Try using a pill organizer, an alarm on your watch or PDA, or a note on the bathroom mirror to remind you to take your preventive medication every day.

Effective Medications for Migraine Prevention

All of the drugs that effectively prevent migraine were originally developed to treat other health problems. The most effective migraine prevention drugs are those that were first used to treat mood disorders, high blood pressure, and epilepsy. Each of these groups of drugs was shown to also reduce migraine headaches when used to treat these other health problems. Only a few medications have received FDA approval for migraine reduction, including timolol (Blocadren), propranolol (Inderal), valproic acid (Depakote), and topiramate (Topamax). Numerous additional medications are widely used to prevent migraine.

Migraine Prevention Medications		
	Typical Dosage	Common Side Effects
Mood Enhancers		
amitriptyline (Elavil)	50–100 milligrams at bedtime	Sleepiness, dry mouth, dizziness, weight gain, constipation. Avoid if you have glaucoma or heart disease.
imipramine (Tofranil)	50–100 milligrams at bedtime	Sleepiness, dry mouth, dizziness, weight gain, constipation. Avoid if you have glaucoma or heart disease.
paroxetine (Paxil)	5–20 milligrams twice daily	Fatigue, loss of libido, weight change.
High Blood Pressure Medications		
timolol (Blocadren)	5–30 milligrams daily	Depression, sedation, constipation, dizziness. Avoid if you have asthma.
propranolol (Inderal)	20–40 milligrams three to four times daily	Depression, sedation, constipation, dizziness. Avoid if you have asthma.
verapamil (Calan, Isoptin)	120–240 milligrams twice daily	Constipation, diarrhea, dizziness, fluid retention.

Epilepsy Medications		
valproic acid (Depakote)	125–250 milligrams twice daily	Tremor, fatigue, hair thinning, weight gain, confusion, menstrual change. Avoid during conception and pregnancy.
topiramate (Topamax)	50–100 milligrams twice daily	Weight loss, nausea, rash, confusion, tingling arms or legs.
gabapentin (Neurontin)	100–400 milligrams two to three times daily	Fatigue, dizziness, decreased appetite.

Preventive medications are initially prescribed in low doses, with the dosage gradually increased over weeks to months to a typical effective dosage. The dosage that will be effective for you may be different from this typical range, depending on other drugs you may be taking, other health problems, and characteristics of your headache. Always review how to take your prescribed medication with your pharmacist or doctor.

WHY TAKE AN ANTIDEPRESSANT IF YOU'RE NOT DEPRESSED?

My doctor gave me an antidepressant for my migraines. I feel like he's not taking my headaches seriously. Why should I take the antidepressant when I'm not depressed?

The same brain chemicals that control migraine, like serotonin, norepinephrine, and GABA, also affect other health conditions. Doctors will often talk about a "chemical imbalance" with depression. Changes in levels of serotonin, norepinephrine, and GABA can influence pain, mood, blood pressure, and risk for seizures. For this reason, the same drug can treat a variety of health problems.

When antidepressants were first tested, treated patients reported improved migraines. Some researchers speculated that antidepressants were reducing migraine because migraine was really a symptom of depression. Interestingly, when levels of depression were measured, migraine activity was just as likely to improve in people who had improvement of their depression as in those whose mood was not improved with the antidepressant (Couch, Ziegler, and Hassanein 1976). This showed that migraine isn't a sign of depression and you can get migraine relief even if you don't have any mood problems.

In the same way, high blood pressure medications can reduce migraines in people with normal blood pressure, and epilepsy medications reduce migraines in people who have never had a seizure. This is because the same chemical messengers that affect migraine can also affect blood pressure in people with hypertension and seizures in people with epilepsy.

WILL TAKING AN ANTIDEPRESSANT MAKE YOU DEPRESSED?

Taking migraine preventive therapy should not cause you to develop problems with depression, high blood pressure, or seizures. Some people have side effects, such as sleepiness, weight change, and dizziness, with daily preventive medications. Some mild side effects may go away after your body adjusts to the new drug. Most side effects go away once the medication is discontinued. Ask your doctor what side effects commonly occur with any medication you're prescribed. If you have these or other side effects, ask your doctor whether you should stop taking this medicine.

HOW DO YOU KNOW WHICH PREVENTION MEDICATION IS RIGHT FOR YOU?

Talk to your doctor to see if you're a candidate for migraine prevention and to determine which treatment will be best for you. Sometimes, migraine prevention therapy can also treat another health problem. For example, people with depression or anxiety plus migraine may be treated with a mood enhancing medication. Similarly, migraineurs with hypertension may be treated with a high blood pressure medication for both conditions.

Unfortunately, finding the right migraine prevention medication usually involves some trial and error. When starting a new migraine prevention medication, you should:

- Make sure you're not overusing acute migraine medications.

- Take your migraine prevention therapy as prescribed every day.

- Monitor your headaches for two to three months.

If one group of medications doesn't work, another might. Possibly, mood enhancing medications won't reduce your migraine, but high blood pressure pills will. Or one epilepsy pill may be ineffective, while another may be very effective. Make sure you try each treatment for at least two to three months before switching to a different pill.

Effective Nonmedication Migraine Prevention

You should consider using nonmedication migraine prevention strategies, even if you are also taking a migraine prevention drug. As with medications, these nonmedication techniques should be used regularly to be most effective.

AVOID TRIGGER EXPOSURE

Review your headache diary to see if you get a migraine at least half of the time after exposure to a particular trigger. If so, you may want to try to minimize your exposure to this trigger. Some triggers can't be avoided, like changes in the weather and menses. Others can be avoided or reduced:

Trigger	Avoidance strategy
stress	• use stress management (see chapter 6)
glare	• add an antiglare screen to your computer • wear sunglasses outside
fasting or skipping meals	• schedule regular meals • have healthy snacks readily available
too much or too little sleep	• maintain a regular sleep schedule
exercise	• stretch before exercise
foods, caffeine, alcohol	• restrict your diet

Eliminate Food Triggers

Both healthy foods (citrus fruits, tomato sauce, peanut butter, and bananas) and junk foods (hot dogs, donuts, and cola) can trigger migraines. These foods contain a variety of chemicals that may trigger migraine nerves in the brain. These chemicals include tyramine, histamine, nitrites, and phenylethylamine. Foods trigger migraines for only about 30 percent of migraineurs (Kohlenberg 1982).

To see if your migraines are triggered by foods, keep a migraine diary while eating your typical diet for one month. Then, for the next month, eliminate all of the following foods:

- aged, cured, or processed meats (hot dogs, sausage, pepperoni, bologna)

- peanuts and peanut butter; pumpkin, sesame, and sunflower seeds

- buttermilk, sour cream, aged "stinky" cheeses

- bananas, strawberries, plums, figs, kiwis, mangoes, raisins, papayas

- tomatoes and tomato sauce, corn, eggplant, pickled vegetables, spinach, sauerkraut, onions, olives, snow peas, beans

- fresh yeast breads, donuts, coffee cake, pizza, sourdough bread

- alcohol, caffeine-containing beverages

- chocolate, mincemeat

- aspartame (an artificial sweetener), monosodium glutamate (sometimes found in Chinese food), canned foods

If a food is not listed above, it's okay to eat.

During this month, keep another headache diary and compare the diary when you eliminated possible trigger foods to the diary when you ate your regular diet. If your headaches are better on the restricted diet, slowly add your favorite foods back into your diet, one food at a time. Notice whether you get a migraine within twelve hours of eating that food. If you do, continue to avoid that food. If you don't, you can resume eating that food.

Eat and Sleep on a Regular Schedule

Avoid skipping meals or fasting. Missing breakfast or lunch is not an effective diet strategy and is likely to make migraines worse. Ideally, you should eat about six times daily, having healthy snacks between meals. Following a structured diet often helps reduce migraines, probably because diets require regularly scheduled meals and snacks.

Try to maintain a consistent sleep pattern, going to bed and rising at similar times every day. If you like to sleep in on the weekends and you get weekend headaches, wake up at your usual (weekday) time. Get up, go to the bathroom, and have a light snack, such as juice and crackers. You can then return to bed. When you get up and have a light snack, your body is able to maintain its regular schedule while you still feel like you're sleeping in.

Add Exercise to Your Daily Routine

Regular aerobic exercise may significantly reduce migraine frequency and severity. In one study, thirty-six migraine sufferers were instructed to do aerobic exercise three times a week for six weeks (Köseoglu et al. 2003). Each session involved ten minutes of warm-up, twenty minutes of aerobic exercise, and ten minutes of cooldown. At the end of the six weeks, migraine frequency decreased by 50 percent, migraine duration decreased by 48 percent, and migraine severity decreased by 33 percent. Brisk walking, biking, and swimming are all good aerobic exercises. Be sure to consult your doctor before beginning any exercise program.

Include stretching in your routine. Stretch twice daily, for around twenty minutes per session. Do stretches slowly, so you feel a normal sensation of stretching but not pain. Hold the stretch for five seconds, relax for five seconds, and then repeat each stretch three to five times. Many stretching exercises can be performed while you're standing or sitting, so you can use them to release stress while sitting in a long meeting or driving, waiting in line at the store, or standing in the shower. Many people stretch while watching their favorite daily television program to increase the likelihood that they will maintain these exercises as part of their daily routine; others stretch before bed to aid sleep.

NECK RANGE OF MOTION. Look straight ahead. Then bend your head forward, moving your chin toward your chest. Hold. Then return to looking straight ahead. Turn your chin toward each shoulder. Then tip your head to each side, moving your ear toward your shoulder. Hold. Then look straight ahead again. Finally, pull in your chin to make a double chin.

SHOULDER SHRUGS. Sit or stand up straight and raise your shoulders straight up. Lower and relax. Then raise your shoulders up and forward. Lower and relax. Then raise your shoulders up and back.

SUBOCCIPITAL RANGE OF MOTION. Drape a bath towel across the back of your neck, with the ends in front of your chest. Gently pull the ends of the towel straight out in front of you, away from your chest. Tilt your chin to your chest. Hold. Then tip your head up and back to look up at the ceiling. Hold. Then tip your head forward to look straight ahead. While looking forward, tilt your head toward each shoulder.

NECK STRETCHES. Tilt your ear toward one shoulder. Keeping your head tipped, tilt your chin forward and toward the opposite side. Gently press your head down toward your chest with your hand to feel a mild stretch in the back of your neck.

NECK ISOMETRICS. Place your palm on your forehead and press your head against it, keeping your palm stationary. Don't let your head or hand move. Repeat with your hand on each side of the head.

HEAD LIFT. Link the fingers of your hands together and hold them behind your neck at the base of your head. Pull your elbows forward and up to achieve the sensation of lifting the head up slightly from the neck.

TURTLE. Look straight ahead and push your chin out in front of you, away from the neck. With your head forward, turn about one inch to each side and then tilt your head about one inch up. Hold for five seconds in each position. Return to facing forward and repeat.

Eliminate Nicotine

You know that cigarette smoking is bad for your health. But did you know that it's also bad for your migraines? Nicotine affects the body's natural pain-fighting chemicals *(endorphins)*, resulting in more discomfort in people with many types of chronic pain, including migraine. One survey of migraineurs showed greater headache severity in cigarette smokers (Payne et al. 1991). Among smoking migraineurs, both headache frequency and severity increased as nicotine use increased. So quitting smoking and getting others around you to quit will probably be good for your migraines as well as your general health.

What Should You Expect from Migraine Prevention?

Use your daily headache diaries to compare migraine activity before and after using migraine prevention. Compare headache severity, duration, and frequency during the month before you began migraine prevention with diaries recorded after you had been using migraine prevention for two to three months. Migraine severity, duration, or frequency should be reduced by half or better. You may also notice the amount of acute migraine medications you need to use is reduced. Use the "Migraine Prevention Satisfaction Assessment" to determine if you have achieved adequate relief.

Exercise: Take the Migraine Prevention Satisfaction Assessment

After using migraine prevention for two to three months, complete this assessment to determine if your preventive therapy is effective.

Prevention treatment: _____

1. Are you having half as many migraines (or fewer) with this treatment?

2. Do the headaches last half as long as they used to or less?

3. Is the severity of your migraines reduced by at least half?

4. Are you using half as many (or fewer) acute migraine pills?

   If you answered yes to any of these questions, your prevention is effective for you. If you are still having frequent or disabling headaches, talk to your doctor about adjusting treatment to try to improve your response. If you're not experiencing effective migraine reduction, talk to your doctor about changing your prevention treatment.

Alternative Migraine Prevention Treatments

I saw a new cure for migraines advertised on television. I know I should be skeptical, but I'm so tired of these headaches. I want a cure!

People have been reporting "cures" for migraines for hundreds of years. Unfortunately, most of the time, a treatment seemed to work for a couple of patients but was later found to be ineffective when tested in large groups of migraine patients. Several alternative therapies have been tested for migraine prevention. Although none of these is a migraine cure, early studies suggest some possible benefits. Botulinum toxin injections, trigger point injections, and acupuncture have all been reported to be helpful in a number of individual migraine patients.

In order to determine if a treatment is really helpful, it needs to be tested in such a way that some patients get the test treatment and other patients get a *placebo*—something that looks like the same treatment but does not include the ingredient that's being tested. The preventive medications discussed earlier in this chapter were all tested in studies in which some patients were treated with the drug and other patients were treated with sugar pills as placebos. Botulinum toxin injections have been compared in studies to injections of plain saltwater. Similarly, acupuncture has been compared with pressing a blunt needle against the skin. Trigger point injections haven't been compared to a placebo treatment in migraine patients. In general, studies haven't consistently shown migraine relief with any of these alternative therapies. Therefore, doctors typically use these therapies as experimental treatments, when other migraine prevention treatments haven't been effective, or when other prevention treatments can't be used due to other health problems.

BOTULINUM TOXIN INJECTIONS

You have probably heard about people getting botulinum toxin (Botox) injections to reduce wrinkles. Botulinum toxin is the poison produced by bacteria in contaminated foods. When you eat food containing botulinum toxin, your muscles—including your breathing muscles—become paralyzed. Untreated botulism causes weakness and even death. This same toxin is injected into muscles of the face and head to temporarily paralyze those muscles, eliminating wrinkles for three to six months. When doctors were doing wrinkle therapy with botulinum toxin, some people reported their migraines also were better for several months. This led to studies investigating botulinum toxin injections for migraine. Two large studies have been conducted in which muscles in the face, head, and neck were injected with either botulinum toxin or a placebo. In one study, migraines were modestly reduced with low-dose botulinum toxin (25 units) but not a higher dose (75 units; Silberstein et al. 2000). In a second study, migraines were no better after injection with either a low (16 units) or high (100 units) dose of botulinum toxin than after injections with placebo (Evers et al. 2004).

TRIGGER POINT INJECTIONS

Some people find that a local injection of a numbing medicine, like novocaine or lidocaine, into the trigger points results in a temporary reduction in migraine (Mellick and Mellick 2003). Trigger point injections are typically only considered in people with a consistently tender muscle area that causes a marked increase in head pain when pressed. Benefits from trigger point injections may last until the numbing medicine wears off (several hours), several days, or rarely several weeks. Trigger point injections should therefore be combined with targeted stretching exercises to help keep muscles loose after the injection wears off.

ACUPUNCTURE

Research investigating whether migraine is reduced with acupuncture has yielded inconsistent results, with benefits in some studies and no benefits in others. In one study, migraineurs treated with acupuncture in addition to their usual migraine treatment experienced about a 30 percent reduction in headache activity, compared to a 15 percent reduction in those not receiving acupuncture (Vickers et al. 2004). A carefully controlled study compared migraine activity in patients who were treated with acupuncture and migraineurs treated with a placebo of a blunt needle pressed against the skin (Linde et al. 2005). In this study, migraine frequency was decreased by at least half in 23 percent of patients treated with the placebo pressure and only 13 percent treated with actual acupuncture.

Preventing Migraine in Women

The same medication and nonmedication treatments that treat migraine in general are also effective for hormonally triggered migraine. Treatment with acute or preventive medications for five to six days, starting three days before the menstrual period, can reduce menstrual migraine. Estrogen therapy may also reduce menstrual headaches. Typical regimens of medications used for migraine prevention around the menstrual period include:

- naproxen: 500 milligrams twice daily
- sumatriptan: 25 milligrams three times daily
- frovatriptan: 2.5 milligrams twice daily
- naratriptan: 1 milligram twice daily
- estrogen: 100 mcg seven-day patch

Before using any of these treatments, discuss them with your doctor.

During pregnancy and breastfeeding, medication options are limited because of concerns for the baby. The same restrictions generally apply to both pregnancy and breastfeeding. Preventive medications that are safe and effective during pregnancy include some high blood pressure medications, like propranolol (Inderal); some antidepressants, like bupropion (Wellbutrin) and paroxetine (Paxil); and gabapentin (Neurontin) in early pregnancy.

Preventing Migraine in Kids

Migraine prevention is essential in children and adolescents with frequent migraines to avoid poor school attendance and academic performance, as well as social isolation from friends. Nonmedication migraine prevention strategies are often helpful in children. Children who consistently experience frequent and disabling migraines may need a daily migraine prevention medication. The mood enhancers amitriptyline (Elavil) and trazodone (Desyrel) and the epilepsy medications valproic acid (Depakote) and topiramate (Topamax) are effective in children and adolescents. Children taking daily migraine medication need to be closely monitored for side effects, especially sleepiness and poor school performance.

6

Manage Your Stress Response

When I talk to my doctor about my migraines, he starts asking if I have any stress. I work full-time and have a daughter in college and two teenagers at home. Of course I have stress! But I still have migraines.

Stress is the most common migraine trigger. Stress *sometimes* provokes a migraine for 50 to 75 percent of migraine sufferers (Marcus 2003b). Only one-third of migraineurs say that stress *usually* triggers a migraine. So stress is only one of many possible triggers for most people. Stress is, however, an important and treatable trigger.

Migraine should not be thought of as a stress problem; rather, exposure to stress may provoke a migraine in people who get migraines. You may be especially susceptible to stress as a migraine trigger on days when you also experience other migraine triggers. For example, Monday may be very stressful at work, but you don't get a migraine. On Thursday, you sleep in, skip breakfast, and feel premenstrual. Stress may then be the straw that breaks the camel's back on this day also filled with other migraine triggers.

Stress Causes Physiological Changes

How many times have you been frustrated when someone asked, "Do you think your headaches are just stress?" While people often think of stress as an emotional problem, it's important to recognize that stress causes a wide variety of physical changes that can aggravate underlying health problems. Exposure to stress causes people with digestive disorders to have diarrhea, diabetics to have poorly controlled blood sugar levels, epileptics to have more seizures, and migraineurs to get more headaches.

When natural disasters occur, you may read reports of the old man who gazes on the devastation of his home, clutches his chest, and drops dead from a heart attack. No one ever says, "Why, that's just a stress heart attack. That doesn't count." Stress precipitated the heart attack, but that was because he already had very bad heart disease. The heart attack was a real physical problem, brought on by the physical changes associated with stress. In the same way, a migraine brought on by stress is just as real as one occurring after you start your menstrual period, eat too many peanuts, or drink red wine.

Exposure to stress may make you feel emotionally anxious, but there are also several physical changes that occur. Think of a day when you're running late for an appointment and you get stuck in traffic. You can feel your teeth clench and jaw muscles tighten. Your neck and shoulder muscles become tense. You'll also begin to sweat. In addition to these changes you can feel, your brain will also begin pumping out pain-provoking chemicals like norepinephrine and dopamine. Stress also affects levels of serotonin and GABA. These chemical changes result in increased migraine susceptibility. So when you're under stress, you may have emotional anxiety, muscle contraction, and brain chemical changes. All of these stress reactions can increase your risk for having a migraine.

You Can Change Your Reaction to Stress

My doctor told me if I got rid of all of my stress, my migraines would be gone.

After hearing that your headaches are "caused" by stress, the next most frustrating suggestion is that you eliminate stresses from your life. Unless you're willing to give up your job, family, friends, and hobbies, you'll probably never eliminate stress. You could eliminate the stress of running late and being stuck in traffic by never making appointments, but that is clearly not reasonable. Instead, you can learn to change your body's response to stress. When you're stuck in traffic, you might normally yell at the car in front of you, clench your jaw, and tighten your shoulder muscles and your grip on the steering wheel. The next time this happens, stop. Take a deep breath. Turn on some soothing music and repeat calming phrases to yourself, like "I will make it to my destination. I am a responsible person. I am prepared for my appointment." In this way, you're not avoiding the stress, but you are changing your physical response to it.

Do You Need Stress Management?

Most migraineurs find that stress will trigger their headaches at least some of the time. Stress management and relaxation therapies are helpful for most people with migraines. To see if stress may be worsening your migraines, take this quiz.

Exercise: Take the Stress Quiz

1. Do at least half of your migraines occur during or after a stressful day?

2. When you get a migraine, do you feel powerless to help yourself get better?

3. Are you so busy with your job and family that you don't have time to do anything else, like hobbies, exercise, or meditation?

4. Do you feel like you're never able to get caught up on your work or chores?

5. Have you had a major life change in the last year (such as change in job, change in family living arrangements, or loss of a close relative or friend)?

6. Do you keep hoping bedtime will come soon so you can finally relax?

If you answered yes to any of these questions, stress may be making your migraines worse. Using stress management and relaxation skills may be an effective way to change your response to stress and reduce your migraines.

Practice Stress Management

My doctor told me to manage my stress. I try not to get upset at things, but the stress is really managing me!

Stress management is not elimination of all stresses. Stress management reduces the body's negative reactions to changes in the environment or other stresses. Both emotional and physical responses to stress can be minimized using strategies such as practicing good time management, identifying your stress buttons, and changing your response to stress.

PRACTICE GOOD TIME MANAGEMENT

Perhaps you, like many people, lead a busy life, scheduling too many activities on a single day. Some unnecessary stress can be reduced by using effective time management. For example, can you do your grocery shopping after you drop the kids off for sports practice rather than making a second trip? Can you carpool with other parents whose kids are participating in the same after-school activities? Can you reduce the number of volunteer activities you do to one or two that are most important to you? Learn to value your time and say no to commitments that will overwhelm your schedule. Don't be afraid to share household chores with your spouse and kids. It's also important for you and your family to have downtime, when no activities are scheduled and you can relax and enjoy each other.

I barely have enough time to brush my teeth in the morning. How can I possibly do twenty minutes of exercise, too?

Trying to fit new migraine-reducing habits into your day may create another stress. Many of the exercises and relaxation techniques in this book can be practiced when you're in the shower, watching television, or waiting in a long line at the grocery store. Using these skills at these times can help fit them into your already busy schedule, and they can serve as stress reducers. You may find that adding a brisk evening walk can be a good way to unwind after a stressful day, get in aerobic exercise, and reconnect with your spouse or teenager if you walk together.

IDENTIFY YOUR STRESS BUTTONS

Learn what situations are stressful for you. For some people, meeting with the boss or speaking in front of a large group is stressful. For others, making a telephone call, waiting in line at the grocery store, talking to your teenager about school, going to the doctor's office, or babysitting a grandchild may be stressful. For many people, fear of getting a migraine is another major stress.

Most people find new situations or changes in usual life patterns stressful. Recognize that even positive change can be stressful: a daughter's engagement, a new baby in the family, or a high school graduation. If you can identify when stress will likely occur, you can take action to prevent a stress response.

CHANGE YOUR RESPONSE TO STRESS

Most people automatically respond to stress by developing a state of excitation: the eyes get wide, the heart races, and muscles get tight. You're ready for a battle. These reactions are helpful when you need to dash to get a boiling pot off the stove or pull a toddler away from the edge of a swimming pool. These same responses, however, can be detrimental in other stressful situations, like taking an examination, talking to your mother-in-law, or presenting a new idea to coworkers.

Stress management asks you to identify stressful situations and change your emotional and physical responses to them. You can minimize the physical effects of stress by:

- recognizing things you can't change (like the weather or your boss's behavior)

- planning for future situations (being prepared reduces stress)

- asking for help

- doing regular aerobic exercise

- practicing relaxation techniques, which will be discussed in detail later in this chapter

WHEN SHOULD YOU USE STRESS MANAGEMENT?

Ideally, you should use stress management strategies before you develop a full stress response. Practice stress management skills before entering a situation that is usually stressful for you. It's easy to see when someone else is "getting stressed." You can watch for those same cues in yourself:

- talking faster or louder than usual
- fidgeting
- racing heartbeat
- tight neck, shoulder, or jaw muscles
- clenching fists

When you recognize that you're beginning to feel stress, take a break and use your stress management skills. Remember, you do not have to eliminate the stress from your environment. You must accept that stress will be around you. However, you can learn to manage your response and avoid the physical changes that can provoke a migraine.

Practice Relaxation and Biofeedback

My doctor told me to relax when I have a migraine. My head's thumping. The lights hurt my eyes. My stomach's upset. How can I relax?

Relaxation techniques are not designed to just make you "chill out" or feel calm. Relaxation techniques are methods to get your brain to decrease chemicals that produce migraine and increase chemicals that protect against migraine. About 60 to 70 percent of migraineurs can reduce their headaches with relaxation techniques (Warner and Lance 1975; Daly et al. 1983). Relaxation techniques can include progressive muscle relaxation, cue-controlled relaxation, and biofeedback. Each of these techniques is described below.

Relaxation techniques are skills that you need to practice to learn. When you first begin, practice them at least five days per week. Each session should last about fifteen to twenty uninterrupted minutes. Sit in a comfortable chair in a quiet room with your arms and legs uncrossed and feet flat on the floor. Close your eyes before you begin.

After you have practiced these techniques regularly for several weeks, you will be able to use them whenever you feel yourself starting to tense or in anticipation of a stressful situation. Relaxation skills can also help reduce pain if you use them when your migraine first begins.

PROGRESSIVE MUSCLE RELAXATION

Progressive muscle relaxation involves tightening and then relaxing different groups of muscles throughout your body. First contract a muscle and hold the tension for ten to fifteen seconds. Then relax this muscle for ten to fifteen seconds. Start with the muscles in your feet. Then contract and relax muscles in this same way in your legs, then your belly, then your arms, then your shoulders, then your neck, then your jaw, then your eyes, and finally your forehead. Pay attention to how each muscle group feels when it is tense and when it is relaxed. With practice, you will begin to notice when your muscles first begin to tighten when you're experiencing stress. For example, you may notice tension in your face, neck, and shoulders when sitting in traffic or waiting in line. Once you feel this tension, work to release it before your migraine develops.

CUE-CONTROLLED RELAXATION

Cue-controlled relaxation uses a combination of deep breathing and repetition of the word "relax." Begin this exercise with a slow, deep abdominal breath. Place your hand over your abdomen to feel it moving in and out with each deep breath. After inhaling, hold your breath for five to ten seconds. Then gradually exhale while slowly repeating (aloud or to yourself) the word "relax." Repeat until your muscles feel loose and relaxed. After you are comfortable with this technique, you should be able to use it before confronting stressful situations, like meeting with the boss, talking to your teenager, or getting a medical test.

THERMAL BIOFEEDBACK

Some people find that it's difficult to "feel" relaxed. *Thermal biofeedback* uses a handheld thermometer to tell you when your body is undergoing the physiological changes associated with relaxation. Place a handheld thermometer between your thumb and forefinger, and measure the temperature. Most people's hand temperature will be between eighty and ninety-four degrees Fahrenheit, or twenty-seven to thirty-four degrees Celsius. Before and after practicing the relaxation skills described above, check your hand temperature. When you become relaxed, the temperature should increase to about ninety-six degrees Fahrenheit or thirty-five to thirty-six degrees Celsius. An inexpensive finger thermometer and biofeedback recording may be obtained from Primary Care Network at (800) 769-7565. Digital biofeedback monitors can be purchased for about twenty dollars. Several companies sell these on the Internet.

Practice Cognitive Restructuring

Cognitive restructuring means that you change the way you think about your migraine. Many people experience *catastrophic thinking,* or assuming the worst, when confronting a stress or a migraine.

Things will never get better.

This pain is never going to go away.

Nothing ever goes right for me.

With this migraine, I'm done for the day.

This thinking presumes that you're powerless to improve your situation. People who engage in catastrophic thinking often believe that the only thing they can do when they have a migraine is to go to bed for the day and be miserable. Over the long run, these negative thoughts can lead to depression, anxiety, and worsened migraines.

Cognitive restructuring teaches you to send yourself more realistic and positive messages when a migraine occurs.

If I use relaxation skills and take my medicine, my headache should improve in an hour or two.

Once my migraine is better, I'll be able to get back to my work.

Even though I have a migraine today, my migraines have been less frequent than they used to be.

Distract Your Brain from the Pain

The brain is very effective at tuning out unwanted messages. If you consider something unimportant, you may ignore it. You've probably had this experience while driving home from work, not really remembering any of the scenery along the familiar route, or tuning out a teacher while you're daydreaming in class. Your brain can also be trained to tune out some pain messages.

Doctors used to advise patients to go to bed in a dark, quiet room as soon as a migraine started. While this may be necessary when the migraine is so severe that you're vomiting, going to a dark, quiet room may actually make the migraine worse. In the dark, quiet room, there is nothing else for your brain to focus on besides the migraine. All of the brain's energy is then devoted to pain messages, which will actually make them stronger since the brain's attention is not being used for anything else. When migraine pain is still mild to moderate, try to distract your brain from the pain by focusing on other things: take a brisk walk, do gentle stretching exercises, practice relaxation techniques, or listen to soothing music. Many people are surprised that their migraine doesn't increase to a full-blown attack when they use these distracting techniques.

Do These Techniques Really Work?

Research studies consistently show that regular use of relaxation techniques results in a 40 to 50 percent reduction in migraines (Holroyd and Penzien 1990; Lake 2001). One study compared headache diaries in migraine patients who were treated with either propranolol as a migraine preventive medication or with relaxation techniques. Migraines were reduced by 43 percent in both groups of patients, with no greater benefit from using the medication than from relaxation techniques (Holroyd and Penzien 1990). Another study compared migraine reduction in patients treated with amitriptyline as a migraine preventive medication compared with stress management. Overall headache activity was reduced by 33 percent with amitriptyline and 58 percent with stress management (Cordingley et al. 1990).

WHY DO STRESS MANAGEMENT AND RELAXATION WORK?

Since I've been practicing stress management and relaxation techniques, my migraines occur less often and they are much more bearable. My husband told me, "See, I told you the migraines were all in your head."

Successful reduction in migraines from stress management does not mean that the migraines were "just a stress problem." Similarly, if relaxation techniques relieve your migraines, this doesn't mean that you had migraines because you were high-strung or anxious. When people develop a sense of control over their stress, their bodies are less likely to release pain-provoking chemicals. In an interesting experiment, Bland and colleagues (2003) found that exposure to a stress that couldn't be escaped resulted in significant changes in brain levels of dopamine and serotonin. If the stress was something that could be escaped, the brain did not change dopamine and serotonin levels. This important study shows that by taking control of your response to stress, you can actually change the likelihood that your brain will send migraine messages. Likewise, using relaxation techniques causes changes in brain serotonin similar to the changes seen with migraine preventive medications (Mathew et al. 1979). These studies show that stress management and relaxation techniques offer much more than just an emotional sense of feeling in control or relaxed. These techniques will actually improve your migraine physiology.

SHOULD I USE STRESS AND RELAXATION TECHNIQUES OR MEDICATIONS?

Stress management and relaxation techniques don't need to replace your migraine medications. Combining migraine medications and relaxation techniques will result in better migraine reduction than using medications or relaxation alone (Holroyd et al. 1995).

Stress Management and Relaxation in Women

Stress management and relaxation are beneficial for headaches occurring with menses, pregnancy, and menopause. They also help reduce reliance on medications during conception and pregnancy. Migraines will naturally improve for about half of women when they are pregnant. This means that migraines won't improve for the other half. Ideally, you should learn these techniques before you begin trying to get pregnant. Headaches improved for 81 percent of pregnant women treated with the combination of relaxation, biofeedback, and physical exercise (Marcus, Scharff, and Turk 1995). This improvement continued throughout the pregnancy and for six months after the baby was born.

Stress Management and Relaxation in Kids

Stress is a common migraine trigger in children and adolescents. They may experience stress related to family situations, school, sports performance, and social relationships. School absence from migraine causes significant stress, because children are concerned about maintaining both academic performance and status in their peer groups. Özge and colleagues (2003) questioned over 500 eight- to sixteen-year-old students with migraine. Migraines occurred on school days for 56 percent of kids. Even though migraines occurred with school, only 16 percent of these kids recognized that school stress was a trigger. Typically, children and adolescents report headaches during the school day, with significant relief of migraines during school vacations, evenings, and weekends. As in adults, this does not mean that children's headaches are imaginary. Children with migraines are just very susceptible to school stress as a trigger.

Stress management and relaxation effectively reduce migraines in kids. In one study, migraines decreased by 53 percent in children and adolescents treated with stress management plus biofeedback (Scharff, Marcus, and Masek 2002). In another study (Sartory et al. 1998), change in migraine was compared in children treated with relaxation plus stress management, biofeedback plus stress management, or migraine prevention medication (metoprolol, a blood pressure medication). Migraine frequency was reduced by 53 percent with relaxation, 54 percent with biofeedback, and 29 percent with medication. Medication use was also reduced by 62 percent in children treated with relaxation and 91 percent in those treated with biofeedback.

Use Vitamins and Herbal Therapies

I'm skeptical about herbal remedies. How can plants possibly help a migraine?

Many medications were originally developed from plants and plant extracts. Native Americans treated pain with willow bark, which was later purified to make aspirin. Similarly, the acute migraine drug dihydroergotamine (DHE) was originally found in a fungus growing on damp rye grain. Today, vitamins, minerals, and herbal supplements are commonly used to treat a variety of health conditions, including migraine. According to Balluz and colleagues (2000), 40 percent of people in the United States had used a vitamin or mineral supplement during the previous month. The use of vitamins and minerals is widespread across the United States for both men and women, all age groups from children to elderly adults, all income levels, and all races and ethnic backgrounds.

Not All Vitamins, Minerals, and Herbs Are Equal for Migraine

You can find rows of vitamins, minerals, and herbal therapies in most grocery stores, pharmacies, or nutrition stores. Only a few of these have been shown to help migraines.

Exercise: Take the Vitamin and Herbal Quiz

Test your knowledge about the use of vitamins, minerals, and herbs for migraine. Which of the following may effectively prevent migraines?

- multivitamins
- vitamin E
- echinacea
- garlic
- bran cereal

Some vitamins and minerals prevent migraines, but they need to be taken in doses much higher than those used in typical daily multivitamins or vitamin supplements. Echinacea is widely used to prevent colds and other infections. Garlic is used to reduce cholesterol and heart disease. Neither of these popular supplements, however, has been identified as a migraine therapy. Interestingly, the only item on the list that may help prevent migraines is bran cereal. Bran cereal contains a high concentration of the mineral magnesium. As you will learn in this chapter, magnesium may be used to prevent migraines.

This chapter will review supplements that are proven migraine preventives. In general, after using these supplements every day for three to four months, you can expect your migraines to decrease by about 25 to 50 percent. So if you normally get four migraines each month, you might get only two or three each month with these treatments. If you normally get eight migraines monthly, your headaches might decrease to four to six attacks each month. Vitamins, minerals, and herbs do not cure migraines completely.

Peppermint oil is the one remedy discussed here that is used as an acute therapy (to treat a headache attack) rather than as a daily prevention therapy. Peppermint oil has not been tested in migraine, but it does reduce tension-type headaches. For this reason, peppermint oil may also be worth trying for migraines.

Vitamins and Minerals

After reading about poor health caused by vitamin deficiency, I started taking vitamin C, vitamin E, and zinc every day. But they don't seem to help my migraines.

With so many vitamins and mineral supplements available, it's important to know which ones may help migraines. Riboflavin, coenzyme Q_{10}, and magnesium are all effective as preventive therapy for migraine. Each of these supplements is considerably more effective than treatment with a placebo. The doses needed to prevent migraine are usually higher than those used for typical health maintenance.

RIBOFLAVIN

Riboflavin, also known as vitamin B_2, is important for turning the foods you eat into energy, for helping to make red blood cells, and for your eyes. Riboflavin is found naturally in dairy foods and green leafy vegetables. The *recommended daily allowance* (RDA) is the amount needed for normal good health. The RDA for riboflavin is 1.1 milligrams daily for women and 1.7 milligrams daily for men. The amount of riboflavin in typical foods is as follows:

- one cup low-fat milk: 0.5 milligrams

- one cup low-fat yogurt: 0.4 milligrams

- half an avocado: 0.2 milligrams

- one-half cup spinach, broccoli, or asparagus: 0.1 milligrams

High doses of riboflavin can be used to prevent migraines. Taking 400 milligrams of riboflavin daily for three months reduces the number of migraine attacks by half (Schoenen, Jacquy, and Lenaerts 1998; Boehnke et al. 2004). Riboflavin doesn't change the severity of the migraines that do occur. In one study, migraine prevention was equally good with either 400 milligrams of riboflavin daily or standard migraine prevention medications (Sándor et al. 2000).

COENZYME Q_{10}

The body makes coenzyme Q_{10}, also called ubiquinone and CoQ_{10}. Coenzyme Q_{10} can also be obtained by eating meats and seafood. Coenzyme Q_{10} is important for metabolism, making energy from food, and boosting the immune system.

Coenzyme Q_{10} taken in doses of 100 milligrams three times daily or 150 milligrams once daily for three months reduces migraine frequency by 27 to 55 percent (Rozen et al. 2002; Sándor et al. 2005). Improvement is better with the 150-milligram daily dose. Very few side effects are reported with coenzyme Q_{10}.

Coenzyme Q_{10} can affect blood sugar metabolism and may change blood clotting. So if you are diabetic or use blood thinners, you should consult your doctor before using coenzyme Q_{10} supplements.

MAGNESIUM

Magnesium is an essential mineral that helps make muscles and nerves work. Magnesium also works as a partner with calcium to build strong bones. Magnesium occurs naturally in whole grains and nuts. The RDA for magnesium is 310 to 320 milligrams daily for women and 400 to 420 milligrams daily for men. The amount of magnesium in typical foods is as follows:

- one ounce roasted pumpkin seeds: 150 milligrams
- one ounce 100 percent bran cereal: 100 milligrams
- one-half cup spinach: 80 milligrams
- one ounce almonds: 80 milligrams
- one ounce dry-roasted peanuts: 50 milligrams
- one-half cup cooked brown rice: 40 milligrams

Magnesium levels in the blood are often low in migraineurs. Taking a 600-milligram magnesium supplement every morning reduces the number of migraine attacks by 42 percent and migraine severity by 34 percent (Peikert, Wilimzig, and Köhne-Volland 1996). The most common side effect is diarrhea, which occurs in 19 percent of migraineurs treated with magnesium.

RECOMMENDED DOSES OF VITAMINS AND MINERALS FOR MIGRAINE

Effective doses of minerals and vitamins for migraine prevention are as follows:

- magnesium: 600 milligrams daily
- riboflavin: 400 milligrams daily
- coenzyme Q_{10}: 150 milligrams daily

Remember that the doses of magnesium and riboflavin that prevent migraine are much higher than the standard doses used in multivitamins. Never take extra doses of multivitamins to achieve the higher doses of magnesium or riboflavin. This would result in dangerously high doses of other vitamins that might make you ill. Always talk to your doctor before using vitamins and minerals.

Herbs

Only a few herbal remedies effectively treat headaches. Feverfew and butterbur root extract are effective for migraine prevention. Peppermint oil may be used to treat an acute headache attack. Each of these treatments is considerably more effective than a placebo.

Always let your doctor know when you are thinking about using an herbal supplement. Some may interfere with prescription or over-the-counter medications. For example, Saint-John's-wort, a popular remedy for depression, should not be used with a triptan medication or prescription antidepressants.

FEVERFEW

Feverfew *(Tanacetum parthenium L.)* is a flower that looks like a daisy. Its main active ingredient is parthenolide. Feverfew reduces inflammation and is commonly used to treat fevers, arthritis, menstrual discomfort, and migraines. Feverfew decreases migraines when taken in doses of 50 to 143 milligrams daily for three to four months (Rios and Passe 2004). With about 100 milligrams of feverfew daily, migraine frequency decreases by 24 percent and migraine severity decreases by 45 percent.

Parthenolide content varies widely among brands of feverfew supplements. A supplement must contain at least 0.2 percent parthenolide to prevent migraines (Rios and Passe 2004). A higher amount of parthenolide (0.5 percent) is available in feverfew manufactured by Galilee Herbal Remedies in Israel. This higher concentration may be more beneficial for reducing migraines.

Feverfew can decrease the ability of the blood to clot. Therefore, people with bleeding disorders should not use feverfew. Do not use feverfew when you are also taking aspirin, anti-inflammatory medications, or other medications that decrease blood clotting.

BUTTERBUR

Butterbur *(Petasites hybridus)* is a perennial shrub. Butterbur root extract (sold under the brand Petadolex) reduces inflammation and is used to treat asthma and migraine. Taking 50 milligrams of butterbur root extract twice daily for three months decreases the number of migraines by 34 to 42 percent (Diener, Rahlfs, and Danesch 2004; Lipton et al. 2004). Migraines decreased by 58 percent when study participants took 75 milligrams butterbur extract twice daily for three months (Lipton et al. 2004). There are very few side effects with butterbur. About one-fourth of migraineurs will experience digestive system side effects, most commonly burping.

PEPPERMINT OIL

Peppermint oil is derived from the plant *Mentha piperita,* with the main active components menthol and menthone. Most people are familiar with peppermint's ability to quiet an uneasy stomach. Peppermint also has painkilling properties. A solution of 10 grams peppermint oil in alcohol may be applied lightly to the forehead and temples. This may be repeated after fifteen and thirty minutes. Peppermint oil reduces tension-type headache pain by 19 percent after thirty minutes and 34 percent after one hour (Göbel et al. 1996). Peppermint oil has not been tested for migraines.

RECOMMENDED DOSES OF HERBS FOR MIGRAINE

Effective doses of herbs for reducing migraines or headaches are as follows:

- feverfew: 100 milligrams containing 0.2 percent parthenolide daily

- butterbur: 50 to 100 milligrams twice daily

- peppermint oil: 10 grams in alcohol applied to the forehead and temples during a headache

Although herbal therapy is often labeled "natural," that does not mean that herbs are free from side effects. Herbal therapy may also interact with other medications you are taking. You should always discuss herbal treatments with your doctor.

Combination Therapy

My mom takes a whole fistful of herbs and supplements every morning for her migraines. Is it necessary or helpful to take so much?

There is little information about using combinations of herbs and minerals for migraine. MigreLief is a product combining 300 milligrams magnesium, 400 milligrams riboflavin, and 100 milligrams feverfew. A study compared migraines in people taking MigreLief and people taking a very low dose of riboflavin (25 milligrams daily) for three months (Maizels, Blumenfeld, and Burchette 2004). Migraine frequency was reduced by about 35 percent with both the combination treatment and the low-dose riboflavin. This suggests that there is no advantage to taking a combination of several natural products for migraine.

Natural Hormones

Melatonin is a natural hormone made by the body to help with sleep. Sleep shuts off serotonin and is a natural remedy for migraine. In one study, taking three milligrams of melatonin thirty minutes before bedtime for three months reduced the number of migraines by 61 percent (Peres et al. 2004). Migraine severity decreased by 51 percent. A few people taking melatonin reported side effects of excessive sleepiness, hair loss, and increased sexual libido. This study needs to be repeated with some participants taking a placebo. These initial results, however, are encouraging.

Vitamins and Herbs in Women

Taking 360 milligrams of magnesium daily for four months has been found to reduce menstrual migraine (Facchinetti et al. 1991). Vitamins and herbs have not been tested for menstrual migraines.

Never take vitamins and minerals (other than your prescribed prenatal vitamin) if you are pregnant or nursing without first talking to your doctor. Feverfew, butterbur extract, and coenzyme Q_{10} should not be used during pregnancy or when you are breastfeeding. Do not use magnesium supplements when you are pregnant.

Vitamins and Herbs in Kids

Few vitamins, minerals, and herbs have been tested in kids and teenagers. Always talk to your doctor before giving vitamin supplements, minerals, or herbs to your child or adolescent.

One large study treated kids and teens with migraine with magnesium for four months (Wang et al. 2003). Magnesium dosage varied according to each child's weight. Magnesium decreased the number of days with migraine by 45 percent. Migraines were also less severe with magnesium. Tension-type headache in children and adolescents may also be substantially reduced with magnesium (Grazzi et al. 2005).

Butterbur root extract was likewise tested in kids and teenagers with migraine (Pothmann and Danesch 2005). Taking 25 to 75 milligrams (depending on the child's weight) of butterbur extract twice daily for four months decreased the number of migraines by 63 percent. Both children and teenagers experienced a similar degree of migraine relief with butterbur. As in adults, the most common side effect was burping.

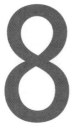

Communicate Effectively

When I try to talk to my doctor about my migraines, I don't even think he's listening to me. He just nods and mumbles, "Um hmm." Then he gives me a new pill to try. Why doesn't he ever just answer my questions?

How many times a day do you feel like someone's not listening to you? It may be your spouse, teenager, or boss—or your doctor. It's easy to become frustrated and angry. When it comes to your migraines, effective communication is essential. If you and your doctor aren't communicating well, you may not get effective treatment. If you're not communicating well with your employer or your family, resentment can build on either side. If your child has migraines, you'll need to work effectively with the school to minimize the impact on your child's education.

Communicating with Your Clinician

When you're talking with your doctor, you may wonder, *Why won't he listen to me? Why doesn't she understand what I'm trying to say? Why don't I understand the terms he's using?* It may surprise you to hear that doctors and other healthcare providers often have these exact same concerns when talking with their patients. We all sometimes feel shy or embarrassed about asking people to repeat or explain themselves. This can be true for both the migraine sufferer and her healthcare provider.

Exercise: Take the Miscommunication Quiz

When you're with your doctor, do find yourself thinking something like this?

- *My doctor never seems to understand what I'm saying.*

- *My doctor's directions are always vague and unclear.*

- *Talking to my doctor is like talking to a wall.*

- *My doctor has the bedside manner of a rock.*

If you typically find yourself leaving your doctor's office frustrated and thinking things like these, you're probably experiencing miscommunication.

RECOGNIZE MISCOMMUNICATIONS

Have you ever said one thing to someone and later found out he interpreted what you said to mean something very different? Miscommunications are a part of everyday life. Unfortunately, miscommunications also frequently occur at the doctor's office. Often, people don't realize that communication is the problem. They may just think their doctor is a cold fish, too busy to listen, or uncaring. Take the miscommunication quiz to see if you might be experiencing poor communication with your doctor.

Notice how poorly this doctor and his patient communicate:

Doctor: Hello, Mary. How are you doing?

Mary: Fine.

Doctor: Anything I can do for you today?

Mary: I guess not.

They didn't say much, but what were they thinking?

Doctor: Are your migraines less frequent with that new pill I gave you?

Mary: Nothing has really changed. I'm still having migraines twice a week, but I don't like to complain.

Doctor: Do you need a treatment change to help get your migraines under control?

Mary: I called the office three times last week and told the nurse how I'm at my wit's end with these migraines. I was hoping you'd suggest something new. I guess I'll just have to learn to live with them.

So the doctor leaves the appointment incorrectly assuming Mary's migraines are well controlled. Mary leaves the appointment thinking there is nothing else that can help her migraines. With better communication, the doctor might have suggested a different treatment. This miscommunication led to poor migraine treatment for Mary.

Mary's doctor didn't ask very good questions. Although Mary can't really change that, she can improve her own communication style to share information with her doctor so she can get better migraine treatment. This chapter will review some easy-to-use techniques you can use to improve communication with your healthcare providers.

DON'T OVERWHELM YOUR DOCTOR WITH QUESTIONS

My doctor told me to write down my questions so I wouldn't forget to ask them. But every time I bring out my notebook, he sighs and slinks toward the doorway.

When your teenager comes to you with a long list of your faults, you may listen to the first one or two, but then you will tune her out. You may start daydreaming: *Is she really serious? How can so many things be that bad?* Your doctor may get the same impression if you try to ask too many questions at each appointment.

You don't have to get a lifetime of questions answered at one doctor visit. Prioritize your concerns and have three or four important questions prepared. Save other questions for another visit, or ask the nurse.

- Select questions that concern you most right now.

  "Are you sure I don't have a brain tumor?"

  "Since I started this pill, I can't sleep and feel confused. Should I keep taking it?"

- Ask questions that need to be answered right away.

  "Will my migraine medicine interfere with a medicine prescribed by another doctor?"

  "Should I take this pill every day or only when I get a migraine?"

- Save questions that can be answered at a later visit.

  "When my daughter has children, will they get migraines, too?"

  "Will my migraines go away once I start menopause?"

Your doctor will be more likely to carefully answer your questions when it's clear they are important and need to be answered at this visit.

COMMUNICATION IS A TWO-WAY STREET

If you and your clinician are having problems communicating, remember that you can help improve this communication. If you don't clearly state your concerns, most healthcare providers will assume that your migraines are no longer a problem, your medications are working well, and you're having no side effects. Ideally, both you and your doctor would be effective communicators. Don't wait for your doctor to improve his communication style. Become a great communicator yourself.

Use Direct and Specific Questions

It is not impolite to ask your doctor specific questions. You'll get the best response when you use clear, direct, and detailed questions. Even though your doctor has treated many people with migraines, he may not know what is most bothersome for you.

For example, if you ask your doctor, "Can people travel with migraines?" he's likely to answer "Yes." This may not be very helpful. When you ask a specific question, you will get a better answer: "I'm concerned about traveling to my daughter's house in Colorado in two weeks. Every time I fly, my migraines get out of control. What can I do to keep my migraines from flaring up when I visit?" Your doctor might suggest using neck stretches during your flight, eating healthy snacks instead of airline peanuts, and drinking extra water when flying. He may also suggest that you try to stay on your regular eating and sleeping schedule. Some people, under their doctor's supervision, even take a water pill to help with migraines that occur with flying or high altitudes. Your doctor probably won't share these practical tips unless you ask a detailed question.

Similarly, if you ask, "What will happen to my migraines when I get pregnant?" your doctor will likely answer, "They'll probably get better." Perhaps what you really want to know is whether you could still take your medications, will the migraines harm the baby, and will you be able to breastfeed. Asking these specific questions would prompt your doctor to explain the risks from your current medications and develop a safe plan for migraine treatment during pregnancy and breastfeeding.

Replace general questions and requests with specific ones.

- Replace "Will this pill help?" with "How long should this pill take to work?"

- Replace "Is this pill safe to take?" with "What side effects should I look for?"

- Replace "I need something for my migraines" with "I'm missing two days of work every week. I need something to knock these migraines out quickly or prevent them from coming."

Share Your Concerns

My headaches are so bad, I can't help but wonder if I have a brain tumor. My doctor doesn't seem worried, though. Is that because I don't have a tumor or he's afraid I'll get upset if he tells me?

Speak up when you have concerns that are not being addressed. Many people's first concern is to make sure their headaches aren't caused by a serious medical condition, like a brain tumor or aneurysm. Their second concern is usually about how to treat the headaches. After examining you, your doctor may think, *These headaches are obviously migraines. There's no sign of a more serious illness.* He may not, however, actually say this to you. Many doctors will simply say, "Here's a pill that should help your migraines." These doctors probably believe that you'll understand the silent message that the headaches aren't caused by something more serious. Doctors are often surprised when patients ask at later visits about getting scans of the brain. These same doctors will often say, "Of course you don't have a brain tumor. I told you these are migraines." They understood that there was no cause for concern about other serious medical conditions, but didn't realize they had not communicated that.

Restate the messages you're hearing from your doctor to make sure you understand. Say things like, "When you said migraine is caused by changes in the brain, does this mean I have a brain tumor?" Or, "When you tell me to take this pill when I get a headache, does that mean I should use it for my mild headaches or just the bad migraines?" Or, "When you said to limit my medications, how many days per week can I use them?" Clarifying what you're hearing is a good way to avoid miscommunication. Restating your doctor's message also reminds your doctor that she needs to provide more specific information to be clearly understood.

Understand Your Treatment Plan

Why did my doctor give me an antidepressant and tell me to see a psychologist for relaxation techniques? I'm not depressed or anxious.

Migraine sufferers often wonder in silence why their doctors prescribed certain treatments. This can be compounded when other people say, "Your doctor doesn't know what he's doing! He gave you a blood pressure pill instead of a headache pill!" or "We told you it was all in your head and you were just depressed." When you don't understand why a treatment is prescribed, you probably won't take it very carefully. Don't be afraid to ask your doctor why a specific treatment was prescribed.

Make Sure Essential Information Is Shared

Make sure you give your doctor complete information about your migraines and other health problems. Migraine information you need to tell your doctor includes:

- how often you get a migraine

- how long your migraine usually lasts

- how disabling your migraine is

- what treatments you have tried in the past

- if you also get other headaches regularly

Make sure you also tell your doctor about:

- other medical conditions you're being treated for

- other health problems you're having

- all of the medications you take

- any other treatment you're getting

When you leave your appointment, make sure you can answer all of these questions:

- What is my headache diagnosis?
- How should I take my medication?
- How long should this medicine take to work?
- What side effects should I watch for?
- When should I make my next visit?

Communicating with Others

Communication with your family, coworkers, and boss is important, too. When you talk with others about your migraines, make it clear that your goal is to develop strategies to minimize the impact of your migraines on others, *not* to get sympathy, request special favors or consideration, or ask to be released from work or household duties.

Most people at least occasionally get a headache, but only about 10 percent of people have disabling headaches. Because of this, most people will believe that your headaches must be mild, just like theirs. If they don't miss school, work, or social events for their headaches, they will be surprised that you need to.

COMMUNICATING AT WORK

I'm really worried about my employee. Once or twice a week, she closes her office door and turns off the lights for a while. Later, when she comes out, she seems kind of spacey. I'm afraid she may have a drug problem.

If your migraines interfere with work, let your boss and affected coworkers know that you get migraines. Also let them know that you're working with your doctor to get an effective treatment to minimize any effects your migraines have on your work. Describe those symptoms that may affect your work:

- "When I have a migraine, I feel dizzy and confused for about fifteen minutes. Then my mind's clear again."

- "When I have a migraine, lights bother my eyes. So it really helps if I can dim the lights."

- "If I take my migraine medication, my headache will be tolerable after about thirty minutes. Then I can get back to work."

If you need to take medicine around coworkers, tell them that you're treating a migraine.

Work with your boss and coworkers to develop strategies that allow you to reduce the impact of your migraines on the work environment. Possible strategies include:

- taking your break early to treat your migraine and working during a later scheduled break

- retreating to a quiet, dim area for thirty to sixty minutes after using your acute migraine treatment

- taking some work home to complete after the migraine resolves

Many employers will make small accommodations when your overall work productivity is good.

Bosses and coworkers don't need to hear about all of your migraine symptoms, how migraines interfere with your home life, or your frustration about having migraines. Work conversations about migraine should focus on reducing work impact.

COMMUNICATING WITH YOUR FAMILY

Remember I have my school play today. I hope you don't get a migraine and miss it.

Migraines can place a strain on family life. Spouses and children may feel guilty, believing that their bad behavior brought on a migraine attack. They may feel angry that migraines keep you from being more involved with them. You may also feel angry at your family's response to your migraines. You may get annoyed when your spouse tries to distract you from your migraine: "Come on, dear. I'm sure you'll feel better once you get moving." You may also feel isolated from your family if they become overly accommodating: "That's okay, Mom. We'll just let you stay home while we go to the museum. You know how the noise and bright lights there can aggravate your headaches." Meanwhile, your family's thinking, *We can't win. She's mad if we include her and mad if we don't. I guess she just expects us to sit around and wait for her to feel better!*

Take time to sit down and talk to your family about your migraines.

- Let your family know that they're not the cause of your migraines.

- Tell your family that you get angry too when you miss out on family activities.

- Talk about ways you can work together to help improve your migraines.

Let your family know that they can help by:

- reminding you to eat and sleep on your regular schedule

- reminding you to do your daily exercise and relaxation

- temporarily doing a chore so you can lie down for thirty minutes after you take your migraine medication

- remembering to include you as part of the family team

COMMUNICATING WITH YOUR CHILD'S SCHOOL

When your child has migraines, it's important that you communicate effectively both with your child and with the school. The most important message your child needs to hear from you is that his job is to do his best in school. Let him know that you understand it's hard to go to school with a migraine. Most migraines can be handled without school absences. Also let him know that you will work hard with him and his doctor to help improve the migraines.

Having migraines in school can be very frustrating for your child. Often school staff, teachers, and fellow students believe children complain about migraines as an excuse to avoid work or tests. Classmates may become resentful that your child gets to stay home from school or go to the nurse, and may begin to tease her about pretending to be sick.

Let your child's principal, teachers, and nurse know that she gets migraines. Describe what symptoms she usually has and how your doctor wants them treated. Be sure to let the teacher know if your doctor wants your child to treat her migraines when they first start, so she'll be allowed to go to the nurse right away. Have medication for your child available at the nurse's office. Develop a plan about how long your child should stay at the nurse's office before returning to class. Migraines in children generally last no more than one to two hours, so most children should be able to go back to class. Watch for how long it takes for your child to start to feel better after treatment. Develop and communicate a plan to both your child and the school. For example, your child may see spots ten minutes before the pain begins. She should go to the nurse at that point and ask for her migraine medication. She may need to lie down for twenty or thirty minutes and do some relaxation exercises. At this point, she may be ready to return to class.

Ask the teacher and school nurse whether your child is requesting to leave class frequently for migraine. If she is, you need to let the doctor know. If your doctor prescribes a daily medication, talk to the teacher to make sure your child's medicine is not making her sleepy in class or harming her school effort.

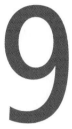

What to Try When Nothing Is Helping

I've seen six doctors, used rows of pill bottles, and listened to a dozen tapes about reducing stress. I don't think anything will ever help my migraines.

It's easy to become frustrated when you get migraines. Although there are a lot of effective treatments available, every treatment doesn't work well for everyone. Most likely you and your doctor will need to try several treatments before finding the one treatment or combination of treatments that works well for you.

If you think that nothing can help your migraines, you're not alone. A large survey of adults with migraine found that about half had not seen their doctor for migraines in the last year (Lipton et al. 2003). Feeling that the doctor couldn't do anything to help the migraines was a common reason for not seeing the doctor. After you've tried a variety of migraine treatments without success, it's easy to feel that there's nothing more to try that will help. Feeling hopeless about your migraines may make you feel helpless, depressed, and frustrated. Don't despair. Remember that there are many effective migraine therapies and researchers are always testing new treatments for migraine.

Make sure you've had a good trial of several usually effective migraine therapies. If you've tried an assortment of treatments without improvement, you may need to talk to your doctor about getting a second opinion from a headache specialist. Remember that your doctor is probably frustrated too. He also wants your migraines to get better. Most doctors will welcome additional opinions and ideas to improve your migraines.

Examine Your Treatment Failures

There can be many reasons migraine treatments haven't worked for you. The fact that several treatments haven't worked doesn't mean that no treatment will ever work. Meet with your doctor to review your previous failed treatments to help develop a strategy for future treatments.

SELECT EFFECTIVE TREATMENTS

My doctor suggested I start taking the same medication my mother used for her migraines. Wouldn't a newer treatment be better?

Some migraine remedies are clearly more effective than others, and some of the most effective treatments have been available for decades. Make sure you have tried a good sample of those treatments that are most likely to be effective. Don't become discouraged if the first several treatments don't help. Migraine treatment is, unfortunately, trial and error. Talk to your doctor about trying a different type of medication if you're still getting frequent or disabling migraines.

ACUTE MIGRAINE MEDICATIONS. The most effective acute migraine medications are analgesics plus caffeine for mild migraines and triptans for moderate to severe migraines (see chapter 4). Try at least three different drugs within each acute medication class before deciding they don't work. So, if one analgesic doesn't work, try a couple of different ones. If one triptan doesn't work, try different brands or formulations (such as nasal sprays or injections).

MIGRAINE PREVENTION MEDICATIONS. The most effective migraine prevention medications are blood pressure medicines, antidepressants, and seizure prevention drugs (see chapter 5). Make sure you have tried at least two different medications in each of these groups. Just because an antidepressant pill didn't work doesn't mean a seizure prevention drug won't work. Your doctor may avoid a group of medications because of your other health problems. For example, people with asthma or low blood pressure may not be able to use some blood pressure medications.

GIVE EACH TREATMENT A GOOD TEST

Make sure you give each new medication a good test. As long as you're not having side effects, stick with the medication long enough to decide if it may work for you.

- Try each acute migraine drug for three different migraines.

- Try each migraine prevention treatment for two to three months.

While you are evaluating a new treatment, make sure you are not taking daily pain medications. Medication overuse is one of the most common reasons for poor relief with acute or preventive migraine therapy (see chapter 2). Migraine treatment won't work if you're regularly using over-the-counter or prescription acute migraine medications at least three days each week. Talk to your doctor about how to reduce excessive use of acute medications.

DON'T EXPECT A CURE

I've tried every pill my doctor has given me, but I'm still getting migraines. Why do I keep getting these awful headaches?

Advertisements have been promising migraine cures for hundreds of years. Although it would be great to find a cure, no available treatment will completely cure your migraines. Don't expect instant relief from acute migraine drugs. Similarly, don't expect that migraine prevention medicine will keep you from ever getting another migraine.

A good response from acute migraine medications is:

- reduction in migraine severity to mild at most after two hours

- reduction in migraine-related disability by at least half

- ability to return to regular activities after two hours

A good response to migraine prevention is:

- reduction in migraine severity or frequency by at least half

- decrease in migraine-related disability by at least half

- no side effects that make you sick or more disabled

Let your doctor know which medications have helped your migraines and what type of relief you need. For example, if a triptan gets rid of your migraine after two hours but you need faster relief, your doctor may suggest switching to a triptan nasal spray or injection. If your migraines occur less often but you're still missing work frequently, your doctor may suggest additional medication or a stronger dose of your prevention therapy.

STICK WITH SUCCESS

I tried doing relaxation exercises, eating regular meals, and exercising for about a month, and my migraines really seemed better. Once I stopped, the migraines were just as bad as they were before treatment. I realized that I have to keep doing those things for them to work.

Once migraines start, they often continue to occur for decades. This means that you'll need to keep using effective treatment for many months or years. When your migraines improve, it's easy to get lazy about watching your diet, keeping up with exercises, and following good stress management strategies. Keep using those treatments that work.

If your migraines are better after you use a migraine prevention medication, your doctor will probably have you continue this medication for at least six months. After that, you and your doctor may decide to try to reduce the dose of your medicine. You may need to go back to a previously effective medication dosage if your migraines increase when you take a lower dose or stop taking the medication.

Reconsider Your Headache Diagnosis

Let your doctor know if your headaches are not improving with treatment. It's possible that you have developed a new type of headache that would need different treatment. Daily headache diaries can help show headache patterns that might suggest a different diagnosis. Keep diaries for two to four weeks. Review these diaries with your doctor to see if your headache pattern or medication use has changed.

Let your doctor know if you develop other health problems. Headaches may be caused or aggravated by a variety of medical conditions, including anemia, thyroid disease, and high blood pressure. Also, let your doctor know if you are taking any new medication or have had a significant change in your life that preceded a worsening of your headache.

Consider Additional Pain Syndromes

Your migraine may be part of a larger chronic pain syndrome. Headache is often associated with changes in the joints or muscles in the neck, shoulders, or spine. Sometimes people don't talk about other body pains because the migraine is what's really bothering them. Other times, they don't mention other pain because they've been told that they shouldn't have pain or that there's nothing that can help with the pain.

Fibromyalgia is a chronic pain syndrome that affects about 2 percent of adults, with women most commonly affected. Fibromyalgia causes widespread pain throughout the body, as well as fatigue, numbness, sleep disturbance, and other physical symptoms. About half of those with fibromyalgia also have migraines (Marcus, Bernstein, and Rudy 2005). Migraines in fibromyalgia patients often don't improve until the fibromyalgia is treated.

See a Headache Specialist

I really like my doctor, but he just keeps trying the same treatments over and over. I don't want to hurt his feelings, but I think I may need a different doctor.

Most family doctors or general practitioners can treat migraines. When migraines don't get better, many people will see a neurologist. For migraines that have not improved, it's often helpful to find a doctor who specializes in treating headache or chronic pain.

Talk to your doctor about seeing a headache specialist if:

- you're still having problematic migraines after several medication trials

- you've been taking the same ineffective treatment for several months

- your doctor says that there are no more treatments to try

Specialty headache or chronic pain clinics are often located at major medical centers. Check with your nearest medical schools for a facility near you. Look for a facility that offers comprehensive services, including a headache specialty doctor, myofascial physical therapists, and pain management psychologists. Make sure the psychologists offer training in pain management skills like relaxation techniques and biofeedback. You can also locate a headache specialist by checking with national headache organizations, like the National Headache Foundation, the American Headache Society, and the American Council for Headache Education. Lists of headache doctors for different geographical regions can be found on the organizations' Web sites (see chapter 10).

10 Get Up-to-Date Migraine Information

*I keep reading about migraine cures. When I try
one of these treatments, it's like taking water.
Am I getting bad information, or are my
migraines just impossible to treat?*

Whenever you hear about a new migraine treatment, your
best resource for reliable information is your doctor.
Before new treatments are made available, they generally undergo years of rigorous testing. During this testing pro-
cess, information about these treatments will be published in
the medical journals that your doctor reads. If your doctor
treats a lot of headache patients, he will probably be very
familiar with most new treatments. You can also find out
about new ways to manage migraine through reliable sources
on the Internet, in books and newsletters, and through
migraine meetings.

Find Reliable Online Information

So many Web sites talk about migraines. How do I know if they're just trying to sell me some new useless remedy or if I can trust what they say?

There's lots of good information and misinformation available on the Internet. If you do a search using the words "migraine treatment," you'll get a list of over 2.5 million Web sites. Even though there are no cures for migraine, a search using "migraine cure" results in almost 700,000 Web sites. You're most likely to find accurate and helpful information on the Internet if you can identify reputable migraine Web sites.

Some of the best sites for reliable and up-to-date information on migraine-related topics are managed by national headache foundations:

- American Council for Headache Education (ACHE) at www.achenet.org
- American Headache Society (AHS) at www .ahsnet.org/ resources/patient.php
- National Headache Foundation (NHF) at www .headaches.org

These sites provide information on testing, diaries, diets, and treatment, as well as specialized topics like migraines in kids, pregnant women, and people with fibromyalgia.

Find Reliable Written Information

Bookstores are full of self-help books on migraine, diet, stress management, and relaxation. These books help supplement your migraine treatment. Don't use self-help books to replace working with your doctor or therapist. You can also find reliable information in newsletters for migraine sufferers. If you find an interesting new treatment or something that makes you question your diagnosis or current treatment, take a copy to your doctor. Sharing your research with your doctor lets her know that you're motivated to get better and willing to try new treatments.

NEWSLETTERS

NHF and ACHE offer migraine newsletters four to six times yearly. These newsletters typically cover a variety of migraine and headache-related topics, including new research and treatments. In each issue, migraine experts from the United States and other countries review the latest headache information and summarize it in terms nonmedical people can easily understand. Previous issues of these newsletters are available for review on each organization's Web site.

RECOMMENDED BOOKS

Look for migraine books that are written by recognized migraine experts. The following books are good resources for additional detailed information on selected migraine topics:

Blumenthal, M., J. Brinckmann, and B. Wollschlaeger. 2003. *The ABC Clinical Guide to Herbs.* New York: Thieme.

Davis, M., E. R. Eshelman, and M. McKay. 2000. *The Relaxation and Stress Reduction Workbook.* Oakland, CA: New Harbinger Publications.

Diamond, S., and A. Diamond. 2001. *Headache and Your Child: The Complete Guide to Understanding and Treating Migraine and Other Headaches in Children and Adolescents.* New York: Fireside.

Sharpe, M. 2001. *The Migraine Cookbook: More Than 100 Healthy and Delicious Recipes for Migraine Sufferers.* New York: Marlowe & Company.

Attend Migraine Meetings and Support Groups

My doctor suggested I go to a migraine support group. What's the use of sitting around and complaining with a bunch of other migraine sufferers? Won't we just make each other even more miserable?

Migraine experts often share new information through meetings and lectures that are directed to people with migraines. Information provided in meetings, lectures, and support groups can keep you tuned in to the latest advances in migraine treatment. Learning about migraines with fellow migraine sufferers can also provide much-needed emotional support and an outlet for your frustrations.

MIGRAINE MEETINGS

Many hospitals and medical schools sponsor health education programs to provide the latest medical information to the public. Check with your local hospital or medical school about the availability of public education programs on migraine. If there isn't one scheduled, put in a request.

MIGRAINE SUPPORT GROUPS

I never knew there were other people who had migraines as bad as mine. I'm sorry they're suffering, but it's nice to know I'm not the only one with bad migraines.

You probably already know lots of people who also have migraines. Many of them may even be in your family. You may not, however, know people who also have severe or frequent migraines. It's easy to feel like something's wrong with you when your migraines seem worse than everyone else's. Support groups provide an opportunity to meet other people who have similarly troublesome migraines. Support groups can also be a good resource for finding out about migraine treatment options in your area.

Both the NHF and ACHE Web sites offer updated listings for local support groups. Select a support group that focuses on positive strategies for migraine improvement. Migraineurs can share where they have found successful treatments, which healthcare providers have been the most helpful, and which treatment strategies have worked for them. Although everyone's migraines are different, talking to others who are struggling with migraines can be a good way to see that you're not alone and that others share your problems and concerns. Many support groups provide a monthly lecture series, which can be a great resource for new migraine information. If you don't have access to a local support group, the NHF provides a service where you can e-mail other migraine sufferers to get their advice and support.

Find the Latest Information About Your Treatment

Your doctor is the best resource for new information about your migraine treatment. You can also ask your pharmacist. The ACHE, AHS, and NHF Web sites are other good resources.

Why is it important to keep up to date about migraine treatment? You've probably noticed that recommendations for diet, exercise, and health maintenance often change over time. What used to be considered harmful is sometimes found to be beneficial. Doctors are still debating whether a little bit of wine is helpful or harmful, how much meat and carbohydrates you should eat, and how much sleep is too much or too little. As new information becomes available, lifestyle recommendations change.

You may be surprised to learn that migraine treatment recommendations evolve, too. With research, doctors learn ways to make treatments more effective. For example, when sumatriptan was first approved, most doctors recommended using a 25-milligram dose. They later learned that migraine sufferers who didn't get relief with 25 milligrams would often get relief with a stronger dose. Unfortunately, many patients who didn't get relief from the low dose never saw their doctors again to try the higher dose. It takes time for doctors to discover what doses and drug combinations work best. It's important to keep learning what's new so you won't miss an opportunity to improve your migraines.

Carefully Judge the Accuracy of Information

Talk to your doctor about new migraine information and treatments. Compare information about new therapies using different resources. For instance, if you hear about a new treatment on television, check out a headache foundation Web site for another opinion.

Be cautious about information that:

- talks about a migraine cure

- recommends you buy a specific product

- recommends a treatment you can only get at one clinic

- sounds too good to be true

- offers a treatment with no side effects

Reliable resources usually offer information about both the benefits and the risks of any treatment. They will also usually discuss other treatment options.

References

Azarbal, B., J. Tobis, W. Suh, V. Chan, C. Dao, and R. Gaster. 2005. Association of interatrial shunts and migraine headaches. Impact of transcatheter closure. *Journal of the American College of Cardiology* 45:489–92.

Balluz, L. S., S. M. Kieszak, R. M. Philen, and J. Mulinare. 2000. Vitamin and mineral supplement use in the United States. *Archives of Family Medicine* 9:258–62.

Beda, R. D., and E. A. Gill. 2005. Patent foramen ovale: Does it play a role in the pathophysiology of migraine headache? *Cardiology Clinics* 23:91–96.

Bland, S. T., D. Hargrave, J. L. Pepin, J. Amat, L. R.Watkins, and S. F. Maier. 2003. Stressor controllability modulates stress-induced dopamine and serotonin efflux and morphine-induced serotonin efflux in the medial prefrontal cortex. *Neuropsychopharmacology* 28:1589–96.

Boehnke, C., U. Reuter, U. Flach, S. Schuh-Hofer, K. M. Einhäupl, and G. Arnold. 2004. High-dose riboflavin treatment is efficacious in migraine prophylaxis: An open study in a tertiary care center. *European Journal of Neurology* 11:475–77.

Boureau, F., J. M. Joubert, V. Lasserre, B. Prum, and G. Delecoeuillerie. 1994. Double-blind comparison of an acetaminophen 400 mg–codeine 25 mg combination versus aspirin 1000 mg and placebo in acute migraine attacks. *Cephalalgia* 14:156–61.

Burstein, R., B. Collins, and M. Jakubowski. 2004. Defeating migraine pain with triptans: A race against the development of cutaneous allodynia. *Annals of Neurology* 55:19–26.

Cordingley, G., K. Holroyd, J. Pingel, A. Jerome, and J. Nash. 1990. Amitriptyline versus stress management therapy in the prophylaxis of chronic tension headache. *Headache* 30:300.

Couch, J. R., D. K. Ziegler, and R. Hassanein. 1976. Amitriptyline in the prophylaxis of migraine. Effectiveness and relationship of amitriptyline and antidepressant effects. *Neurology* 26:121–27.

Daly, E. J., P. A. Donn, M. J. Galliher, and J. S. Zimmerman. 1983. Biofeedback application to migraine and tension headache: A double-blind outcome study. *Biofeedback and Self-Regulation* 8:135–52.

Diener, H. C., V. W. Rahlfs, and U. Danesch. 2004. The first placebo-controlled trial of a special butterbur root extract for the prevention of migraine: Reanalysis of efficacy criteria. *European Neurology* 51:89–97.

Evers, S., J. Vollmer-Haase, S. Schwaag, A. Rahmann, I. W. Husstedt, and A. Frese. 2004. Botulinun toxin A in the prophylactic treatment of migraine: A randomized, double-blind, placebo-controlled study. *Cephalalgia* 24:838–43.

Facchinetti, F., G. Sances, P. Borella, A. R. Genazzani, and G. Nappi. 1991. Magnesium prophylaxis of menstrual migraine: Effects on intracellular magnesium. *Headache* 31:298–301.

Gerth, W. C., G. W. Carides, E. J. Dasbach, W. H. Visser, and N. C. Santanello. 2001. The multinational impact of migraine symptoms on healthcare utilisation and work loss. *Pharmacoeconomics* 19:197–206.

Göbel, H., J. Fresenius, A. Heinze, M. Dworschak, and D. Soyka. 1996. Effectiveness of Oleum menthae piperitae and paracetamol in therapy of headache of the tension type. *Nervenarzt* 67:672–81.

Grazzi, L., F. Andrasik, S. Usai, and G. Bussone. 2005. Magnesium as a treatment for paediatric tension-type headache: A clinical replication series. *Neurological Sciences* 25:338–41.

Hamalainen, M. L., K. Hoppu, E. Valkeila, and P. Santavuori. 1997. Ibuprofen or acetaminophen for the acute treatment of migraine in children: A double-blind, randomized, placebo-controlled, crossover study. *Neurology* 48:103–7.

Holroyd, K. A., J. L. France, G. E. Cordingley, L. A. Rokicki, S. A. Kvaal, G. L. Lipchik, and H. R. McCool. 1995. Enhancing the effectiveness of relaxation–thermal biofeedback training with propranolol hydrochloride. *Journal of Consulting and Clinical Psychology* 63:327–30.

Holroyd, K. A., and D. B. Penzien. 1990. Pharmacological versus non-pharmacological prophylaxis of recurrent migraine headache: A meta-analytic review of clinical trials. *Pain* 42:1–13.

Honkasalo, M-L., J. Kaprio, T. Winter, K. Heikkilä, M. Sillanpää, and M. Koskenvuo. 1995. Migraine and concomitant symptoms among 8,167 adult twin pairs. *Headache* 35:70–78.

Kelman, L. 2004. The premonitory symptoms (prodrome): A tertiary care study of 893 migraineurs. *Headache* 44:865–72.

Kohlenberg, R. J. 1982. Tyramine sensitivity in dietary migraine: A critical review. *Headache* 22:30–34.

Köseoglu, E., A. Akboyraz, A. Soyuer, and A. Ö. Ersoy. 2003. Aerobic exercise and plasma beta endorphin levels in patients with migrainous headache without aura. *Cephalalgia* 23:972–76.

Krymchantowski, A. V., and J. S. Barbosa. 2002. Rizatriptan combined with rofecoxib vs. rizatriptan for the acute treatment of migraine: An open label pilot study. *Cephalalgia* 22:309–312.

Lake, A. E. 2001. Behavioral and nonpharmacological treatments of headache. *The Medical Clinics of North America* 85:1055–75.

Lance, J. C., and A. S. Arciniegas. 2002. Post-traumatic headache. *Current Treatment Options in Neurology* 4:89–104.

Lewis, D., S. Ashwal, A. Hershey, D. Hirtz, M. Yonker, and S. Silberstein. 2004. Practice parameter: Pharmacological treatment of migraine headache in children and adolescents. Report of the American Academy of Neurology Quality Standards Subcommittee and the Practice Committee of the Child Neurology Society. *Neurology* 63:2215–24.

Linde, K., A. Streng, S. Jurgen, A. Hoppe, B. Brinkhaus, C. Witt, S. Wagenpfeil, V. Pfaffenrath, M. G. Hammes, W.

Wiedenhammer, S. N. Willich, and D. Melchart. 2005. Acupuncture for patients with migraine: A randomized controlled trial. *Journal of the American Medical Association* 293:2118–25.

Lipton, R. B., and M. E. Bigal. 2005. Migraine: Epidemiology, impact, and risk factors for progression. *Headache* 45 (suppl. 1): S3–S13.

Lipton, R. B., H. Göbel, K. M. Einhäupl, K. Wilks, and A. Mauskop. 2004. *Petasites hybridus* root (butterbur) is an effective preventive treatment for migraine. *Neurology* 63:2240–44.

Lipton, R. B., A. I. Scher, T. J. Steiner, M. E. Bigal, K. Kolodner, J. N. Lieberman, and W. F. Stewart. 2003. Patterns of health care utilization for migraine in England and the United States. *Neurology* 60:441–48.

Luciani, R., D. Carter, L. Mannix, M. Hemphill, M. Diamond, and R. Cady. 2000. Prevention of migraine during prodrome with naratriptan. *Cephalalgia* 20:122–26.

Maizels, M., A. Blumenfeld, and R. Burchette. 2004. A combination of riboflavin, magnesium, and feverfew for migraine prophylaxis: A randomized trial. *Headache* 44:885–90.

Marcus, D. A. 2003a. Central nervous system abnormalities in migraine. *Expert Opinion on Pharmacotherapy* 4:1709–15.

Marcus, D. A. 2003b. Chronic headache: The importance of trigger identification. *Headache and Pain* 14:139–44.

Marcus, D. A., C. Bernstein, and T. E. Rudy. Forthcoming. Fibromyalgia and headache: An epidemiological study supporting migraine as part of the fibromyalgia syndrome. *Clinical Rheumatology*.

Marcus, D. A., L. Scharff, and D. C. Turk. 1995. Nonpharmacological management of headaches during pregnancy. *Psychosomatic Medicine* 57:527–35.

Mathew, N. T., J. Kailasam, P. Gentry, and O. Chernyshev. 2000. Treatment of nonresponders to oral sumatriptan with zolmitriptan and rizatriptan: A comparative open trial. *Headache* 40:464–65.

Mathew, R. C., B. T. Ho, P. Kralik, and J. L. Claghorn. 1979. Biochemical basis for biofeedback treatment of migraine: A hypothesis. *Headache* 19:290–93.

Mellick, G. A., and L. B. Mellick. 2003. Regional head and face pain relief following lower cervical intramuscular anesthetic injection. *Headache* 43:1109–11.

Miller, D. S., C. A. Talbot, W. Simpson, and A. Korey. 1987. A comparison of naproxen sodium, acetaminophen and placebo in the treatment of muscle contraction headache. *Headache* 27:392–96.

Mortelmans, K., M. Post, V. Thijs, L. Herroelen, and W. Budts. 2005. The influence of percutaneous atrial septal defect closure on the occurrence of migraine. *European Heart Journal* doi:10.1093/eurheart/hei170.

Neri, I., F. Granella, R. Nappi, G. C. Manzoni, F. Facchinetti, and A. R. Genazzani. 1993. Characteristics of headache at menopause: A clinico-epidemiologic study. *Maturitas* 17:31–37.

Özge, A., R. Bugdayci, T. Sasmaz, H. Kaleağasi, Ö. Kurt, A. Karakelle, H. Tezcan, and A. Siva. 2003. The sensitivity and specificity of the case definition criteria in diagnosis of headache: A school-based epidemiological study of 5,562 children in Mersin. *Cephalalgia* 23:138–45.

Packard, R. C. 1992. Posttraumatic headache: Permanency and relationship to legal settlement. *Headache* 32:496–500.

Payne, T. J., B. Stetson, V. M. Stevens, C. A. Johnson, D. B. Penzien, and B. Van Dorsten. 1991. Impact of cigarette smoking on headache activity in headache patients. *Headache* 31:329–32.

Peikert, A., C. Wilimzig, and R. Köhne-Volland. 1996. Prophylaxis of migraine with oral magnesium: Results from a prospective, multicenter, placebo-controlled and double-blind randomized study. *Cephalalgia* 16:257–63.

Peres, M. P., E. Zukerman, F. da Cunha Tanuri, F. R. Moreira, and J. Cipolla-Neto. 2004. Melatonin, 3 mg, is effective for migraine prevention. *Neurology* 63:757.

Peroutka, S. J., J. A. Lyon, J. Swarbrick, R. B. Lipton, K. Kolodner, and J. Goldstein. 2004. Efficacy of diclofenac sodium softgel 100 mg with or without caffeine 100 mg in migraine without aura: A randomized, double-blind, crossover study. *Headache* 44:136–41.

Pothmann, R., and U. Danesch. 2005. Migraine prevention in children and adolescents: Results of an open study with a special butterbur root extract. *Headache* 45:196–203.

Rapoport, A. M., R. E. Weeks, F. D. Sheftell, S. M. Baskin, and J. Verdi. 1986. The "analgesic wash-out period": A critical variable in the evaluation of treatment efficacy. *Neurology* 36 (suppl. 1): 100–101.

Reisman, M., R. D. Christofferson, J. Jesurum, J. V. Olsen, M. P. Spencer, K. A. Krabill, L. Diehl, S. Aurora, and W. A. Gray. 2005. Migraine headache relief after transcatheter closure of patent foramen ovale. *Journal of the American College of Cardiology* 45:493–95.

Rios, J., and M. M. Passe. 2004. Evidence-based use of botanicals, minerals, and vitamins in the prophylactic treatment of migraine. *Journal of the American Academy of Nurse Practitioners* 16:251–56.

Rozen, T. D., M. L. Oshinsky, C. A. Geneline, K. C. Bradley, W. B. Young, A. L. Shechter, and S. D. Silberstein. 2002. Open label trial of coenzyme Q_{10} as a migraine preventive. *Cephalalgia* 22:137–41.

Sándor, P. S., J. Áfra, A. Ambrosini, and J. Schoenen. 2000. Prophylactic treatment of migraine with â-blockers and riboflavin: Differential effects on the intensity dependence of auditory evoked cortical potentials. *Headache* 40:30–35.

Sándor, P. S., L. Di Clemente, G. Coppola, U. Saenger, A. Fumal, D. Magis, L. Seidel, R. M. Agosti, and J. Schoenen. 2005. Efficacy of coenzyme Q_{10} in migraine prophylaxis: A randomized controlled trial. *Neurology* 64:713–15.

Sartory, G., B. Muller, J. Metsch, and R. Pothmann. 1998. A comparison of psychological and pharmacological treatment of pediatric migraine. *Behavior Research and Therapy* 36:1155–70.

Schachtel, B. P., S. A. Furey, and W. R. Thoden. 1996. Nonprescription ibuprofen and acetaminophen in the treatment of tension-type headache. *Journal of Clinical Pharmacology* 36:1120–25.

Scharff, L., D. A. Marcus, and B. J. Masek. 2002. A controlled study of minimal-contact thermal biofeedback treatment in children with migraine. *Journal of Pediatric Psychology* 27:109–19.

Schoenen, J., J. Jacquy, and M. Lenaerts. 1998. Effectiveness of high-dose riboflavin in migraine prophylaxis: A randomized controlled trial. *Neurology* 50:466–70.

Schreiber, C. P., S. Hutchinson, C. J. Webster, M. Ames, M. S. Richardson, and C. Powers. 2004. Prevalence of migraine in patients with a history of self-reported or physician-diagnosed "sinus" headache. *Archives of Internal Medicine* 164:1769–72.

Silberstein, S., N. Mathew, J. Saper, and S. Jenkins. 2000. Botulinum toxin type A as a migraine preventive treatment. *Headache* 40:445–50.

Stone, A. A., J. E. Broderick, S. S. Shiffman, and J. E. Schwartz. 2004. Understanding recall of weekly pain from a momentary assessment perspective: Absolute agreement, between- and within-person consistency, and judged change in weekly pain. *Pain* 107:61–69.

Vickers, A. J., R. W. Rees, C. E. Zollman, R. McCarney, C. M. Smith, N. Ellis, P. Fisher, and R. Van Haselen. 2004. Acupuncture for chronic headache in primary care: Large, pragmatic, randomised trial. *British Medical Journal* 328:744.

Wang, F., S. K. Van Den Eeden, L. M. Ackerson, S. E. Salk, R. H. Reince, and R. J. Elin. 2003. Oral magnesium oxide prophylaxis of frequent migrainous headache in children: A randomized, double-blind, placebo-controlled trial. *Headache* 43:601–10.

Warner, G., and J. W. Lance. 1975. Relaxation therapy in migraine and chronic tension headache. *Medical Journal of Australia* 1:298–301.

Welch, K. M., V. Nagesh, S. K. Aurora, and N. Gelman. 2001. Periaqueductal gray matter dysfunction in migraine: Cause of the burden of illness? *Headache* 41:629–37.

Wojnar-Horton, R. E., L. P. Hackett, P. Yapp, L. J. Dusci, M. Paech, and K. F. Ilett. 1996. Distribution and excretion of sumatriptan in human milk. *British Journal of Clinical Pharmacology* 41:217–21.

Dawn A. Marcus, MD, is associate professor in the Departments of Anesthesiology and Neurology at the University of Pittsburgh School of Medicine. She is a neurologist with the Pain Evaluation and Treatment Institute in Pittsburgh and coordinator of the institute's Interdisciplinary Headache Clinic. She is an active member of the American Pain Society and the American Association for the Study of Headache. She has received research grants to investigate various issues in headache, including headaches in pregnant women and the mechanisms of recurring headaches.

Some Other
New Harbinger Titles